SAMe*
(*S-adenosylmethionine)

The European
Arthritis and
Depression Breakthrough

SOL GRAZI, M.D.
MARIE COSTA

PRIMA HEALTH
A Division of Prima Publishing

Warning—Disclaimer

This book is not intended to provide medical advice and is sold with the understanding that the publisher and the author are not liable for the misconception or misuse of information provided. The author and Prima Publishing shall have neither liability nor responsibility to any person or entity with respect to any loss, damage, or injury caused or alleged to be caused directly or indirectly by the information contained in this book or the use of any products mentioned. Readers should not use any of the products discussed in this book without the advice of a medical professional.

The Food and Drug Administration has not approved the use of any of the natural treatments discussed in this book. This book, and the information contained herein, has not been approved by the Food and Drug Administration.

Library of Congress Cataloging-in-Publication Data

Grazi, Sol.
    SAMe (S-adenosylmethionine) : the European arthritis and depression breakthrough / Sol Grazi and Marie Costa.
        p. cm.
    Includes index.
    ISBN 0-7615-1627-1
    1. Adenosylmethionine—Therapeutic use.   2. Osteoarthritis—Alternative treatment. 3. Depression, Mental—Alternative treatment.
I. Costa, Marie.   II. Title.
    RM666.A278G73   1998
615'.36—dc21
                                                    98-34443
                                                    CIP

99 00 01 02 03 HH 10 9 8 7 6 5 4 3 2
Printed in the United States of America

How to Order
Single copies may be ordered from Prima Publishing, P.O. Box 1260BK, Rocklin, CA 95677; telephone (916) 632-4400. Quantity discounts are also available. On your letterhead, include information concerning the intended use of the books and the number of books you wish to purchase.

Visit us online at www.primahealth.com

This book is dedicated to Gino Pedicino,
in gratitude for his unique perspective
and intuitive knowledge
that ours would be a partnership made in heaven.

Acknowledgments

Even though this book is written in my voice for the sake of clarity, it is actually a duet and not a solo. Therefore I humbly and gratefully acknowledge my partner, Marie Costa.

I would also like to thank my sister and family practitioner par magnifique Margie, for her efforts in ensuring that the information in this book is both high quality and contemporaneous; my daughter Lila, who has done so many things to further the book's production, and whom I wish the best of luck in her own medical career; and, as always, my wife Martha, who balanced the work, anxiety, and trauma of writing a book with her kind devotion, attention, and patience.

CONTENTS

INTRODUCTION

Remember Juan Ponce de Leon, the sixteenth century Spanish explorer who was looking for the Fountain of Youth and instead discovered Florida? From our "modern" almost twenty-first century view, such a quest seems hopelessly deluded, even amusing. But despite our superior knowledge and technology, we aren't a whole lot different from poor old Juan. We're still looking for that magical fountain, although it has changed form somewhat. Now youth comes in the form of a pill you can swallow, a potion you can inject, drops you can put on your tongue, or a cream you can rub on your skin. Retin-A, vitamin E, antioxidants, growth hormones—it seems as though every month we hear about another discovery that promises to restore vitality, erase wrinkles, vanquish aches and pains, tone muscles, and extend life. Many substances even go beyond these claims. We hear that they can prevent cancer and heart disease, jump-start a flagging libido, melt off unwanted pounds, and increase mental alertness and capacity. And of course all of this takes very little effort (though likely considerable expense) on our part.

If you think I sound skeptical, you're right. I don't believe there is any substance, natural or otherwise, that has the power to bestow health and youth, at least not all by itself. I tend to take a conservative approach to manipulating body chemistry, because in spite of all our scientific knowledge, there is so much more that we don't know about the incredibly complex and wondrous workings of the human body.

That's why I initially had some doubts about a supplement with the unlikely name "Sam," which was supposedly working wonders for Europeans with conditions as diverse as osteoarthritis, depression, heart disease, Alzheimer's disease, migraines, and cirrhosis of the liver. But I was intrigued enough to take a closer look at Sam, otherwise known as S-adenosylmethionine (ess-add-eh-NO-sil-meth-EYE-uh-neen), or SAMe. What I saw impressed me enough that I changed my mind and agreed to write this book, with the caveat that it would be as balanced and objective as I could make it.

SAMe is the latest in a long line of drugs and supplements being marketed to a public anxious for relief from a wide variety of illnesses and afflictions. Some of these substances have been developed by honest scientists motivated by a thirst for knowledge and a desire to benefit humankind. Others have been concocted by charlatans looking to make a quick buck. Some are unquestionably beneficial. Some have the potential to harm as well as help. Some are both harmless and ineffective, and a few harm without helping. The challenge for the concerned physician or suffering patient is to determine where on this spectrum a given substance falls. If it falls into the first two categories, then the question is whether it can benefit a specific individual, and at what risk.

Unfortunately (except for those who profit by it), the all too human desire for a quick fix—preferably with as little effort and change as possible—leads many people to jump on the latest supplement bandwagon without weighing the potential risks and benefits. We've seen it happen with L-tryptophan, melatonin, and DHEA, which are all naturally produced substances that have become available in supplement form. We've also seen it happen with herbs such as echinacea and St. John's wort. While many people, including respected medical researchers and scientists, believe that some or all of these can help at least some people some of the time, none of these supplements is the long-sought after panacea that will cure all human ills.

And neither, I can say quite definitively, is SAMe. It won't cure everything that ails you, and it won't make you immortal or restore your lost youth. But SAMe does have some remarkable properties that may make it helpful for some common conditions that have resisted conventional treatment. In fact, the more I learn about SAMe, the more bewildered I am that something so obviously beneficial is not already in common use in this country as it is overseas. I suspect that once word gets out, it will become quite popular. Therefore, my job is to make sure that potential beneficiaries, as well as those whom SAMe probably *won't* help, have access to the information they need to make smart decisions about it.

CHAPTER 1

WHAT IS SAMe?

S-adenosylmethionine, or SAMe, is a substance that is synthesized from the amino acid methionine and that is found literally everywhere in the body. In biochemical terms, SAMe is a "methyl donor." It carries a very important piece of a molecule that is critical to a myriad of body processes, such as making cartilage, detoxifying blood, and regulating mood. SAMe works within the cell, stimulating biochemical reactions that transform various "raw materials" into bioactive substances that the body can use, such as neurotransmitters, DNA, RNA, and protein.

In the mid-seventies, Italian scientists developed a form of exogenous SAMe (exogenous means that it is produced outside the body). Since then, the supplement, also known as S-adenosyl-L-methionine, ademetionine, or AdoMet, has been credited with slowing or reversing the progress of osteoarthritis, improving memory, alleviating depression, and reducing alcohol-induced liver damage, among other feats. As word of SAMe's apparent healing properties spread, so did its popularity. In many parts of Europe, particularly in Italy, SAMe is now an accepted part of modern medical treatments.

Riding the wave of its European popularity and a flurry of enthusiastic media reports on its presumed benefits, SAMe is likely to be touted as the next surefire remedy for a wide range of conditions, including some for which it has no confirmed effect.

But can SAMe live up to its hype? The answer is a qualified "maybe." If even half the reports about it are true, it has the potential to be an effective treatment for at least one—and possibly several—of the most common ailments that afflict modern humankind. If research in the United States affirms what Europeans have found in studies involving over 20,000 people, it will be shown to have few, if any, serious side effects. And if widespread use turns up no new indications of toxicity, it will be one of the safest treatments presently available for osteoarthritis and depression, as well as some types of heart disease and liver ailments.

In short, if SAMe keeps its promise, it may prove to be of greater benefit than many modern high-tech drugs that are far more expensive, if not in actual cost, then in terms of treating their side effects and toxicity. SAMe could be among a variety of substances, such as insulin, that are both indigenous to our bodies and provide treatment for what ails us.

If It's So Great, Why Haven't You Heard of It?

If SAMe is potentially so useful, you are probably wondering why you haven't heard of it before. The short answer is, I don't know. But the reasons may lie, to a large extent, in the workings of the American medical machine and the American psyche.

Long ago, in a *Saturday Night Live* skit, Steve Martin, playing the part of a medieval doctor, explained that his patient's ailment would have once been thought to be caused by evil spirits. But modern knowledge, he declared, had determined it was the result of a small dwarf in the patient's stomach. The catalog of human knowledge still contains many such dwarves. Even the best scientists are limited by the "known facts" and prejudices of their times. For instance, it wasn't that long ago when doctors used bloodletting to treat a wide variety of ailments ranging from headache to gout. As our knowledge of the human body and its workings has grown, so has our ability to evaluate the effectiveness of such remedies. As a result, most people consider bloodletting a relic of bygone times, although it is still considered an appropriate therapy for a handful of rare conditions, including hemachromatosis, a disorder in which iron accumulates in the blood and organs, and polycythemia vera, a disease that causes an overaccumulation of red blood corpuscles.

At the same time, other treatments once dismissed as old-fashioned or barbaric are coming back into use because their effectiveness has been proven even to confirmed skeptics. For example, leeches long symbolized the crudeness and ignorance of medieval medicine. Yet they are now becoming the treatment of choice for restoring blood circulation to grafted tissue and reattached appendages, such as ears, fingers, and toes. Additionally, leech saliva contains anticoagulant and clot-digesting compounds that may soon be used to make drugs for treating cardiovascular diseases such as heart attacks and strokes.

Sometimes modern medicine takes traditional or folk remedies and refines them to increase and expand their effectiveness. An example of this is foxglove, an herb that has long been used to bring down the swelling of edema, which happens when excess fluid accumulates in the cells. Scientists eventually isolated the active substance in foxglove as digitalis. They determined that it reduces edema not by acting as a diuretic, or "water pill," but by improving the pumping function of the heart, enabling it to move blood more effectively and thus keep fluid from backing up into body tissues. As a result of this discovery, digitalis is now commonly used to improve cardiac function in people with heart failure.

If even half the reports about [SAMe] are true, it has the potential to be an effective treatment for at least one—and possibly several—of the most common ailments that afflict humankind.

Despite such strong evidence that healers of olden times did not function wholly from superstition and ignorance, members of the American medical establishment have historically been resistant to so-called natural and herbal remedies. In Europe, however, attitudes are different, which is why options such as St. John's wort and SAMe found their first supporters overseas. Although western and central Europe was the center of modern medicine for several centuries, the Europeans have continued the close connections to their roots in traditional healing. This has enabled them to maintain a more open stance towards supplements and other modes of healing outside the conventional western model. Both France and Germany maintain formal scientific, social, and political connections to homeopathy, naturopathy, chiropractic, and other healing endeavors. Thus, their scientists are more willing to conduct research in these arenas, and their governments are more willing to fund such research. In this environment, approaches that would be considered alternative in the U.S. are accepted modes of treatment in European countries. German doctors, for example, are more likely to prescribe St. John's wort than Prozac for depression.

Americans, on the other hand, have tended to lean heavily on the scientific model and to trust more in technology than in natural forms of healing. In the nineteenth century, the first "regular" medical doctors fought hard and long to gain dominance over the illegitimate sellers of patent medicines. The battle continued into this century, where it has focused on more legitimate—but philosophically different—disciplines such as chiropractic and homeopathy. Until recently, most American medical practitioners had a tough time even partially accepting healing events and processes that did not fit into the conventional western model. This has been especially true in the schools where new physicians learn the art and science of their profession.

Ironically, faith in the effectiveness of conventional medical science is not necessarily more grounded in reality than many of the claims for so-called alternative medicine. It is true that we don't have solid scientific explanations for why acupuncture, tai chi, and chicken soup help people heal, although millions of people swear that they do. However, it is also true that we don't really know why many conventional treatments work, including such common ones as aspirin and antidepressants. Even more ironic, many accepted medical treatments do not hold up any better under rigorous studies than either alternative remedies or placebos.

Whether in recognition of these truths, out of frustration with the inability of conventional medicine to deal effectively with their suffering, or simply from a desire to explore every possibility, Americans are turning to alternative therapies in ever-increasing numbers. The growing availability of medical information in the media, bookstores, and on the Internet— much of it admittedly of questionable value—has also prompted people to seek out remedies on their own. More and more people try therapies, herbs, or supplements based not just on the recommendations of their doctors, chiropractors, or naturopaths, but on the advice of friends, neighbors, and coworkers.

This consumer-led movement is fostering a growing recognition among medical professionals that many so-called alternative treatments are at least as effective as conventional ones and are often cheaper and less risky. As a result, fissures are beginning to appear in the wall erected between conventional and alternative medicine, and there are signs that the wall may soon collapse altogether. Many doctors, particularly younger ones, actively seek information on nutritional supplements and various alternative therapies and recommend them to patients. Most medical insurance plans cover at least some chiropractic care, and many cover massage therapy for certain conditions. HMOs are conducting yoga, nutrition, and stress reduction classes. Half of American medical schools now offer one or more courses dealing with alternative medicine. The Food and Drug Administration (FDA) is permitting investigative studies of herbs and supplements for treating specific conditions. The publishers of the *Physicians' Desk Reference* (PDR) are putting out monographs on herbs. And major pharmaceutical companies are spending millions of dollars to research, develop, and test herbal and supplement formulas that can be patented and/or approved by the FDA as medical treatments.

In this environment, SAMe is bound to find a receptive market. Like other natural supplements, it appeals to people who care about the substances and foods they put in their body. Unlike a drug, per se, SAMe is not a foreign molecule with the ability to attach to a receptor and displace what would naturally go there. Rather, it is an intimate part of the body's metabolic mechanism, without which the body works poorly, if at all. Exogenous SAMe fits right in with native SAMe, not displacing it, but augmenting it to further stimulate its natural function.

One factor that is probably both a cause and a result of SAMe's relative anonymity is that, until recently, it has been relatively difficult to find in the United States. In addition, some domestic sources charge very high prices for SAMe, which they attribute to their high cost to obtain and package it and the as yet small demand. Whether a surge of public interest in SAMe will have the effect of expanding availability and reducing cost remains to be seen.

Is SAMe Safe?

SAMe's safety may be its most potent advantage. All the available evidence seems to indicate that SAMe's toxicity is about as close to zero as possible. This fact alone could make it the treatment of choice for a number of conditions, since all of the drugs currently in use for those conditions have severe drawbacks in terms of both short-term side effects and the potential for long-term harm.

When scientists talk about the toxicity of a substance, they are referring to its ability to damage specific organs or systems of the body. The question is, what kind of and how much damage does it do? I often say that as a doctor, I deal in poisons. This is because, at some level, all medicines are poisons. The data on any drug always includes a report of its toxicity, and that level is nearly always something other than zero. Many common drugs are potent poisons indeed—at least to some people.

. . . members of the American medical establishment have historically been resistant to so-called natural and herbal remedies. In Europe, however, attitudes are different, which is why options such as St. John's wort and SAMe found their first supporters overseas.

This point was underscored by a study that recently appeared in the *Journal of the American Medical Association (JAMA).*

The study was a meta-analysis—that is, it reviewed the results of many small studies to arrive at an overall finding. The study's authors estimated that anywhere from 76,000 to 137,000 hospital deaths each year are the result of adverse drug reactions. Another 2.2 million people suffer nonfatal adverse reactions. These reactions do not occur as a result of patient misuse or doctor error. They are simply caused by an individual's bad reactions to proper doses of prescribed drugs. Everyone's physiology is unique, and it's nearly impossible to predict how a given person will react to a specific drug—even one that the majority of people tolerate well.[1]

So why use drugs at all? Because they help people. Overall, far more people benefit from legally prescribed drugs than are harmed by them. For example, curare is a deadly poison, but its muscle relaxing properties make it effective for anesthesia. Chemotherapy literally poisons the body in an often successful attempt to kill the invading cancer. Narcotics, which can provide blessed relief from unbearable pain, can cause respiration to slow down or even stop altogether, leading to brain damage or death.

The truth is, any substance is poisonous in sufficient quantities. Even water can be a poison that when inhaled keeps lungs from obtaining oxygen, leading to death. Natural carcinogens are all around us—in the food we eat and the air we breathe. Living on earth is a constant exercise in balancing our poisons. As a doctor, the questions I must continually ask are: "Are the poisons I use safer or more beneficial than not using poisons at all? When is a given poison appropriate, and in what doses?" Sometimes, the cure is literally worse than the disease. Other times, the right amount of the right kind of poison can drive away disease and give a body a chance to heal.

Fear of toxicity has kept many potentially helpful drugs off the market in the United States, primarily because of the FDA's dedication to keeping Americans from consuming anything that remotely might be harmful. Lest we put the entire blame on the FDA, however, it should be noted that Americans in general tend to have an attitude that simultaneously says, "if a little is good, then more is better" and "if some is bad, any is terrible." This has led to cultural and governmental craziness (like the Alar apple scare of a few years ago), along with misguided and doomed attempts to reduce the level of carcinogens in foods and the environment to zero.

As noted above, however, there are indications that the FDA is easing up on its resistance to new or imported drugs, and particularly, that it is opening up avenues for approval of herbal formulas and supplements to treat specific conditions. The FDA has approved the sale of SAMe in this country. However, as a nutritional supplement, SAMe is classified as a food, not as a drug. This means that it has not gone through the rigorous testing and clinical trials required for FDA approval of drugs. To receive FDA approval as a nutritional supplement, a substance must simply meet minimal standards of safety; that is, it must be fairly evident that it doesn't hurt or kill people. The manufacturer is not required to show that the supplement produces any health benefits—nor can it claim that it does. Unfortunately, the manufacturer is also not obligated to ensure a supplement's purity and consistency—or even to guarantee that the tablets, capsules, or liquid in a bottle actually contain the substance named on the label.

That said, what is known about SAMe seems to indicate an almost complete lack of toxicity. The available studies are admittedly sparse. In a 1988 study done on pregnant rats, there was no damage to the fetus at doses more than ten times the maximum recommended human dose. A comparable study on rabbits showed no problems at doses similar to those recommended for humans.[2] In a later study, rats showed no chromosomal damage even at doses as high as fifty times the maximum human dose.[3]

Unlike a drug, per se, SAMe is not a foreign molecule with the ability to attach to a receptor and displace what would naturally go there. Rather, it is an innate part of the body's metabolic mechanism, without which the body works poorly, if at all.

What side effects did occur in these studies were transient (temporary). They included local tissue reaction at the site of injection and slowed body weight gain (which some people would consider a benefit). High intravenous doses sometimes resulted in rigidity and shortness of breath. In another study, in which SAMe was injected directly into the brains (something that is unlikely to be done to humans), the rats developed Parkinson's-like symptoms with a corresponding brain chemical pattern similar to that of a person with

Parkinson's disease. These symptoms included tremors, rigidity, abnormal posture, and dose-related hypokinesia, or decreased ability to move.[4] SAMe may also have an adverse effect on the ability of cytosine arabinoside (an anti-cancer agent) to inhibit cancer cell growth.[5] These effects are minor compared to the effects of drugs that SAMe would augment or replace, such as anti-inflammatories and antidepressants.

Does SAMe Work?

Many Europeans, both doctors and patients, believe that SAMe works. As we shall see, support is strongest for its effectiveness in treating osteoarthritis, either alone or in conjunction with other drugs or supplements such as glucosamine. The evidence is somewhat less strong for its value in treating depression. There is also evidence that SAMe reduces liver damage in the presence of acute and chronic toxins, most significantly alcohol.

All the available evidence seems to indicate that SAMe's toxicity is about as close to zero as possible.

SAMe is also being used for other problems, some of which lack a known pharmaceutical response. Among these is fibromyalgia, in which SAMe is supposed to reduce muscle pain and improve fatigue. There is even a report or two of beneficial effects on Alzheimer's disease. These responses, if valid, could be a function of SAMe's action on the blood vessels, or another as yet undetected process.

Will SAMe Work for Me?

Ah, that is the question. And I can't answer it for sure—no one can. But this book will explore what is known about SAMe, what it may be able to do for various conditions, and how we think it might work. It will then give you some guidelines for deciding whether to try SAMe yourself, as well as looking at how you can integrate SAMe into a healing strategy that includes lifestyle factors and other conventional and alternative treatments. Once we've completed our exploration, you will be better equipped to determine whether SAMe can support your healing, or will turn out to be just another expensive and time-consuming side trip on your journey to health.

CHAPTER 2

UNDERSTANDING SUPPLEMENTS

upplement is probably one of the most misunderstood words in medicine. At its broadest, the term refers to a substance that is naturally used or produced in the body, and that is used to supplement or augment existing body processes. But this definition is rather misleading, as we shall see. In this chapter, I'll attempt to clear up some of this misunderstanding, so you will have a better picture not only of SAMe, but of the whole array of supplements and how they are used, misused, and even abused. We'll start by looking at the most common and familiar supplements—the co-enzymes.

Co-Enzymes:
Vitamins, Minerals, and Fatty Acids

As we will see later, our bodies and all other living things are in essence chemical factories. At any given instant, your body is carrying on countless chemical reactions that allow it to perform myriad functions, including:

- Metabolizing food and oxygen

- Generating thoughts and emotions

- Contracting and relaxing muscles

- Detoxifying dangerous substances

- Growing and dividing cells

Because these reactions take place at a molecular level, far from where we experience our mind and body, we tend to not give them much thought. Truly, however, they are one (or many) of nature's wonders.

If you've ever taken a course in chemistry, especially organic chemistry, you'll recall that many chemical reactions can take place only in extreme conditions involving either pH (acid concentration), osmolality (the concentration of particles in water), temperature, or all three. When scientists generate reactions in a laboratory, the pH can range from extremely acidic (pH 3, for example, sulfuric acid) to extremely alkaline (pH 8 or 9, for example, lye), while temperatures can range from almost freezing to boiling. The particle concentration can reach a supersaturated level where the particles precipitate (separate) into a solid within the water. An example of a supersaturated solution is the grade school experiment in which you make rock candy by suspending a string in a mixture of sugar and water. The sugar crystals precipitate onto the string (fun on a string—not so much fun in a blood vessel). Obviously, if these conditions occurred in a living body, the body would not stay living for long. And even if it were possible for the body to engineer and survive such extremes, regulation would be an insoluble dilemma, for you could not simultaneously have reactions requiring, for example, a 33-degree and a 120-degree environment.

Enzymes are organic catalysts, able to cause, within a very narrow range of environments, reactions that would ordinarily require extremes of pH, osmolality, or temperature to occur.

Enter enzymes. Enzymes are organic catalysts, able to cause, within a very narrow range of environments, reactions that would ordinarily require extremes of pH, osmolality, or temperature to occur. In the body, the "climate control setting" is an average pH of 7.4, with a range that goes down to about 7.2 and up to 7.7. Go beyond these boundaries in either direction and you have, as they say, one sick puppy (or person). In a healthy human, the temperature range is two degrees either side of normal (98.6 degrees). Even in someone who is ill, the range is perhaps 90 to 106 degrees. Again, step outside that range and your chances of survival are marginal at best.

Enzymes can cause chemical reactions to occur within a tiny range of pH—7.4 plus or minus 0.1—and a temperature of 98.6 plus or minus two degrees. These little packets of reaction facilitators cannot work alone, however. They need other substances to help them along. The general term for these helper substances is co-enzymes. Co-enzymes found in the body include vitamins, minerals, and some kinds of fatty acids. Each of these molecules plays a role in helping enzymes perform their function.

Our first indirect evidence of the existence of co-enzymes came in 1757, when an English physician named Lind discovered a way to prevent scurvy, a connective tissue disease that primarily affected British sailors. Previously, deficiency disorders had been seen only in people who were starving, so it was believed that the starvation itself caused the various symptoms. Lind, however, theorized that scurvy was a result of something missing from the sailors' diets. The sailors made an ideal study group for testing this hypothesis since they were separated from the rest of the English public by virtue of their long isolation at sea. Lind compared the sailors' diets with those of their landlubber countrymen, and determined that the difference was a lack of citrus fruit and green leafy vegetables, neither of which was a staple of shipboard life. Citrus fruit was not native to their homeland, and green leafy vegetables spoiled too quickly to be carried on board (refrigeration had not yet been invented). Lind solved the problem by suggesting that the sailors include limes as a regular part of their diet, thus giving rise to the sobriquet "limey."

It wasn't until the 1930s that a scientist named Szent-Györgi discovered the molecular structure for vitamin C, which was the actual substance that was missing in the sailors' diet of hardtack and canned pork (or whatever British sailors actually ate). Shortly thereafter, scientists determined vitamin C's actual function as a co-enzyme in collagen synthesis. This discovery led to the identification of several other molecules that the body uses in various chemical reactions but does not produce itself. These became known as vitamins. Finding vitamins in various foods made it possible to conduct empirical experiments in which specific vitamins were eliminated from subjects' diets. The resulting diseases indicated the significance of the vitamin being studied. Through these studies, researchers identified diseases associated with specific vitamin deficiencies. Beriberi, for example, results from thiamine deficiency, and pellagra is caused by a lack of niacin. A lack of vitamins A, D, B6, riboflavin, and pantothenic acid can also result in well-defined disorders.

In addition to vitamins, the body requires certain minerals to keep its chemical factory going. Magnesium, calcium, and phosphorus are necessary for healthy bones and muscles. Iodine is needed for proper thyroid function. Sodium and potassium are essential for conducting nerve impulses and contracting muscles. Important trace minerals—so-called because they are needed only in minute amounts—include copper, selenium, and zinc.

The Essential Amino Acids

Amino acids are the building blocks of proteins. Proteins are the organic molecules that perform a wide range of body functions. Among the many types of proteins are enzymes—the organic catalysts mentioned above that guide chemical reactions.

Some amino acids can be synthesized by the body. The remainder must be supplied by diet; these are called the essential amino acids. Humans have 11 essential amino acids, including cystine, tyrosine, lysine, methionine, and tryptophan.

One source of essential amino acids is the protein found in foods such as meat, eggs, and soybeans.

One source of essential amino acids is the protein found in foods such as meat, eggs, and soybeans. In the digestive tract, food protein is broken down into its amino acid components, which cells then use to synthesize other proteins that the body needs. However, not all protein sources are created equal. Some 20 years ago, starvation diets became popular as people tried to lose maximum weight in minimal time. The result was a rash of deficiency disorders. At the time, a researcher named George Blackburn was studying hospitalized patients who were essentially starving after having surgery (particularly abdominal surgery), which precluded them from eating until their bowels had regained normal function. The researcher found that the patients were losing muscle mass due to a protein deficiency. In essence, their bodies were raiding their own muscles for protein. He discovered that the deficiency could be mitigated by giving the patients an average of four ounces of protein a day.

As all too often happens, scientific research evolved into popular myth, resulting in a new diet that caught the fat-conscious public by storm—the protein sparing modified fast (PSMF). Unfortunately, the market response to this demand was to offer a protein powder derived from horse hooves, which was an unbalanced source of protein that was missing several of the essential amino acids. Sadly, a number of the people using the powder ended up in intensive care units with abnormal heart rhythms. In some cases the rhythm never reverted to normal, and the dieters died.

Subsequent research revealed that the bizarre diet was lacking a whole array of important substances in addition to the amino acids. Those substances included potassium, calcium, phosphate, and magnesium, as well as five trace minerals: cobalt, chromium, copper, manganese, and selenium. In a normal diet, these substances are easily obtained in the minute quantities required. The PSMF diet was modified to include the missing substances and is now relatively safe. Like other fasting-oriented diets that have come and gone over the years, however, it is still neither wise nor particularly effective, especially if the goal is lasting weight loss.

Supplements Used to Enhance
Natural Body Processes

In addition to the co-enzymes and essential amino acids, there is another group of supplements that are less easy to categorize. This group consists of substances that are either naturally used or made by the body and that can be augmented in order to enhance an already occurring process. This is called "loading the system." You can think of it in terms of a chemical equation with different substances on either side. The substance on the left side is the precursor, which, through a chemical reaction or series of reactions, is transformed into the substance on the right side of the equation. If you load the system with additional amounts of the precursor substance, the body produces more of the resulting substance in order to balance the equation.

An example of a precursor is L-tryptophan, one of the essential amino acids from which the neurotransmitter serotonin is made. Supplementing the body's supply of L-tryptophan results in increased serotonin production. Clinically, this translates to feelings of relaxation in a statistically significant percentage of people. Unfortunately, as described in Chapter 9, the FDA removed L-tryptophan from the market in 1989, because certain batches of it included a highly toxic substance that caused a potentially fatal disease called eosinophilic myalgia syndrome (EMS). Other examples of supplements used to load the system in order to enhance desirable processes are glucosamine and SAMe.

Supplement or Drug?

As I've defined it here, the general category of supplements includes:

- Co-enzymes, such as vitamins and minerals

- Essential amino acids

- Certain other substances that occur naturally either in the environment or in the body itself

This definition is still somewhat less than satisfactory, as it seems to include substances that also occur naturally in the body, but that are generally regarded as drugs in their exogenous form (e.g., insulin, thyroxine, and steroids). One difference is that these substances have been approved by the Food and Drug Administration (FDA) for treating specific conditions. There are some reports that SAMe is currently being investigated as a treatment for cirrhosis of the liver and possibly other conditions as well. If it gains such approval, it may slip over into the category of "drug." So perhaps the final part of our definition, in this country at least, is that supplements are sold over the counter and are not closely regulated by the FDA. The same criteria could be used to separate "herbs" from those "drugs" that are derived from plant sources.

I suspect that in many cases, the supplement versus drug dichotomy is as much political and emotional as actual. If people are opposed to conventional medical practices for whatever reason, using herbs and supplements appears to be a reasonable alternative approach. It's certainly a profitable one. The market for herbs and supplements is growing at a phenomenal rate, though it has yet to match the multi-billion dollar pharmaceutical industry.

I have heard rumors that the major drug companies are becoming interested in entering the supplement market. Additionally, the FDA is looking for ways to exert some control over the production and marketing of herbs and supplements. These changes could have both positive and negative implications for consumers. On the plus side, they could alleviate what is perhaps the biggest problem with herbs and supplements—the lack of enforceable standards.

The FDA imposes strict standards on drug manufacturers that sell their products in this country. These include a recognizably measured and consistent amount of the drug, consistent bioavailability (the drug is made in a form that is available to or readily absorbed by the body), and the absence of extraneous or dangerous fillers.

> *Most vitamins are manufactured, rather than being extracted from natural substances, and there is every reason to think that they work just fine in the body.*

Unfortunately, there are no similar controls in the supplement industry. This means you have no way, short of running your own chemical tests, to be sure of what you are buying. This is especially true of herbs, since individual plants vary greatly in the concentration and the purity of the substances they contain, and few companies test the plants before processing them. Other types of supplements are not immune to this problem, however, as evidenced by the contaminated L-tryptophan batches. Another example is the sale during the late seventies and early eighties of calcium-magnesium supplements made from minerals that were abundantly available. Unfortunately, the minerals contained enough lead that a person taking the pills over a period of time would sustain lead poisoning.

A related problem is the lack of standard dosages. Most people take herbs and supplements based on the recommendations of store clerks, few of whom are even remotely qualified to give good advice. Even if they were qualified, the aforementioned problem with purity and strength makes getting a consistent dose next to impossible. Added to this is the tendency among many people to think that if a little is good, more is better—an approach that can be expensive and sometimes dangerous, particularly with some of the more potent herbs.

The downside to herbs and supplements being produced and marketed by major pharmaceutical companies and regulated by the FDA is that they may become both less available and more expensive. We could also see certain products become completely unavailable if they happen to compete with more profitable drugs. I believe this is, in part, what happened with L-tryptophan, and it could certainly happen with SAMe.

"Natural" versus Manufactured

One reason people take supplements is that they believe the supplements are more "natural" and thus, by implication or assertion, preferable to drugs. However, many supplements, including SAMe, are manufactured versions of their naturally occurring counterparts. Most vitamins are manufactured, rather than being extracted from natural substances, and there is every reason to think that they work just fine in the body. This does not stop people from paying premium rates for the so-called natural versions, in the belief that their bodies can tell the difference. For example, producers and consumers of vitamin C extracted from natural sources, such as rose hips, insist that it is superior to the manufactured version because it contains other molecules similar to vitamin C, called flavonoids. Although that argument may be tempting, there isn't any solid evidence to back it up.

Similarly, the vast majority of doctors who prescribe thyroid medications for patients choose a manufactured form called levothyroxine (or Synthroid), rather than thyroid extract, which comes from sheep. The reason for this is that the levothyroxine is more easily measured, and its effects are the same in 99 percent of cases. I have a few patients who believe that the extract works better for them than levothyroxine, but I think this is primarily a matter of perception. They think that natural is better, so for them it is.

The fact is, if a substance is bioactive—that is, if it has an effect on the body—it is bioactive whether it is natural or manufactured. Taking too much of a natural supplement is as dangerous as taking too much of a manufactured one. On the other hand, if a substance is always benign, it is less likely to have an effect on the body at all, in which case its use is superfluous.

Why or Why Not Take Supplements?

All of the substances I've mentioned so far are required for normal body functioning. They are also either naturally produced by the human body or present in food and/or water. Whether it is necessary for healthy people to supplement their diets with additional amounts of these substances is a subject of some controversy.

Supplement manufacturers, along with natural foods retailers and mail-order suppliers, have profited handsomely by responding to the supposed deficiencies created by processed food—an environment perceived by many as toxic—and people's desire to be smarter, more energetic, and eternally youthful. Marketers have been phenomenally successful at convincing people that they need to take substances that either have always been missing in the normal human diet, or have been leeched out during the time it takes food to get from the point of production to the dinner table. By this argument, even fresh fruits, vegetables, and meats are suspect. After all, how much nutrition can be left in a banana that has traveled by boat from El Salvador to Savannah, and then by truck to the regional distributor, before arriving at your local supermarket? This marketing approach works, in part, because it connects universal symptoms such as mild fatigue, headaches, and a host of other vague ills to these supposed deficiencies. Compelling as the argument may be, scientists have yet to prove any connection between the modern diet and the myriad symptoms that, I suspect, past generations accepted as a fact of life.

In theory, people who eat a regularly balanced diet should be able to obtain all of the substances that are not naturally made in a healthy body.

In theory, people who eat a regularly balanced diet should be able to obtain all of the substances that are not naturally made in a healthy body. Many supplements may be at best superfluous (since the body uses only as much of a given substance as it needs) and at worst harmful (since many substances, including several vitamins, can become toxic if you get too much of them). Nonetheless, I would be hesitant to state definitively that there are no benefits to taking daily vitamins to replace those that have been depleted from the so-called fresh fruits and vegetables found in the supermarket. There just isn't enough scientific evidence at this point to justify either taking vitamins or refraining from taking them.

Supplements like SAMe are most likely to be effective if you have a condition that the supplement supports, such as osteoarthritis, liver disease, or depression.

One way to reduce the possibility that the foods you eat will be vitamin-deficient is to take the macrobiotic approach. This means eating fresh foods that come from the same latitude where you live and preferably from the same region. Purchasing and consuming foods close to where they are produced greatly reduces the chances of vitamin depletion due to age and travel. Eating a balanced diet, especially in this way, should meet most people's need for vitamins and trace minerals.

On the other hand, there are times when the body needs some extra help, and supplements makes sense. Many diabetics, for example, would die without an external source of insulin. Persons with hypothyroidism can benefit greatly from taking Synthroid or thyroid extract. On a less dramatic level, I have often been able to relieve patients' leg cramps by adding potassium to their diets. Similarly, zinc supplements are beneficial for acute or chronic prostatitis, relieving pain and swelling as well as improving function and strength.

Supplements like SAMe are most likely to be effective if you have a condition that the supplement supports, such as osteoarthritis, liver disease, or depression. Simply having low ambient levels of SAMe is *not* a reason to take it. As we will see, some conditions associated with low SAMe levels, such as Parkinson's disease, did not improve with SAMe supplementation.

CHAPTER 3

WEIGHING THE
EVIDENCE

I n this book, we will examine the evidence about SAMe in order to address some key questions:

What is SAMe's nature?

What are the issues involved with it?

What beneficial and/or harmful effects has it shown, if any?

In the process, we will compare SAMe with other substances used to treat various conditions. For osteoarthritis, we'll compare SAMe with the anti-inflammatories, and for depression, we'll compare it with various types of antidepressants. For liver disease and cirrhosis conventional medicine has no effective treatment, so there won't be much to compare with SAMe.

You will have the task of assessing the evidence and determining whether SAMe has any potential value for you. This chapter provides some guidelines for evaluating the available information and deciding whether or not you should try SAMe, or for that matter, other treatments that have been touted in the media or recommended to you by a practitioner, friend, or health food store employee. This applies to both conventional and so-called alternative remedies. As I explained in the last chapter, I do not consider SAMe an alternative drug per se, because the term "alternative" is more of a political and social label than anything related to real science. Like any drug or supplement, either SAMe has merit or it doesn't, and it should be judged on its effectiveness and potential for harm, not on its perceived naturalness or lack thereof.

Understanding Correlation
and Cause and Effect

Almost all medical science is based on correlation, because the world is much too complex to let us isolate all the possible causes for a given effect. In fact, we are coming to a different understanding of how both our bodies and the world as a whole work. Rather than living in a world of simple cause-and-effect relationships—like the one germ, one disease theory—we are coming to understand that any given event involves a number of different factors whose preponderance creates a critical mass that leads to that event. Take, for example, a plane crash. The reason it takes the National Transportation Safety Board months, or even years, to analyze a crash is that there is almost never one clear cause. Instead, there is a build-up of factors which, when combined at a particular place and time, result in the plane crashing.

In the same way, every disease is the result of multiple, largely unknown factors including:

- Genetic susceptibility

- Psychological orientation

- Environment

- Occupation

- Exposure to pathogens, and more

For example, the type of body a person has, her metabolism, the strength of her muscles, and the work she does on a daily basis may all contribute to her developing osteoarthritis. Changing just one of these factors may be enough to prevent the disease process from occurring.

Does the fact that we cannot discern direct causes and effects mean we should be suspicious of all the processes and therapies that we've been working with? Of course not. If a treatment works for a significant percentage of people, and does minimal harm, then it has a positive effect.

The Hazards of Searching for Cause-and-Effect Relationships

Because cause-and-effect relationships are so imprecise, it is easy to see correlations that may not actually exist. A glaring example of this has to do with the supposed relationship between cholesterol levels and heart disease. For decades, the American medical establishment and the public at large have "known" that high cholesterol levels can lead to coronary artery disease. Billions of research dollars have been spent trying to corroborate this assertion and develop therapies for reducing the risk attributed to high cholesterol. But even when it first came out, the correlation was not that clear. Over the years, a number of different meta-studies (see below for a definition of a meta-study) have examined the cholesterol–heart disease correlation. It is less than reassuring to know that many of them do not agree with the general consensus. Here are a couple of examples:

- "Screening with total cholesterol levels is most likely to be useful when done in populations at high short-term risk for dying of coronary heart disease. In other populations, the benefits of reduction are much smaller or are uncertain."[1]

- "Primary prevention trials, however, generally have failed to show a beneficial effect of cholesterol lowering on total mortality, because of both low overall death rates and a disturbingly high number of deaths from non-coronary causes."[2]

This is not the only example of suspect correlations that have entered the popular realm as accepted truth. In the early 1970s, when coronary care units (CCU) were first becoming popular, researchers discovered that over 50 percent of the people who came into CCUs for first-time myocardial infarction did not have *any* of the risk factors commonly accepted for heart disease.[3] A World Health Organization (WHO) study at around the same time compared risk factors for heart disease in Parisians with those in the United States. As it turned out, Parisians had all of the risk factors in abundance. They ate greasy foods and exercised less than Americans. Their cholesterol levels were significantly higher. They drank more and smoked a lot more. Yet, surprisingly, they had a lower incidence of heart disease.

. . . we are coming to a different understanding of how both our bodies and the world as a whole work. Rather than living in a world of simple cause-and-effect relationships—like the one germ, one disease theory— we are coming to understand that any given event involves a number of different factors whose preponderance creates a critical mass that leads to the event.

This news led American researchers to seek a substance that might be cardioprotective and that would account for the reduced incidence of heart disease in the French as compared to Americans. They came up with the astounding conclusion that the tannin in red wine was the differentiating factor.

When this report hit the media, sales of red wine increased exponentially in this country. However, the increased consumption of tannin did not lead to a corresponding decrease in coronary artery disease. So perhaps the researchers were off the mark in their analysis.

All of this means we need to be very careful when we observe correlations that may suggest cause and effect. A cause and effect that is clearly established is one that occurs every single time. For instance, if I move a light switch up and the light goes on, and I move the switch down and the light goes off, and I do that a hundred times and get the same effect each time, I can deduce that there is a direct cause-and-effect relationship between my moving the switch and the status of the light. If I move the light switch up and the light goes on some of the time, there may be a correlation between the two. Or there may be just a random association, and the two events aren't really connected at all. To help determine the likelihood that a direct correlation exists between two processes, scientists use another tool, called statistics. The purpose of statistical analysis is to determine whether an event occurs more often than would happen by mere chance. If it does, we say that it is statistically significant.

Understanding Types of Evidence

There are two major types of evidence related to the effectiveness of medical treatments:

- Anecdotal
- Scientific

The stronger of the two, by far, is scientific evidence, although anecdotal reports can be of value if you take into account their limitations. Let's consider some of the ways that we can make sense out of the information that we get from both types of evidence.

Anecdotal Evidence

Anecdotal evidence includes testimonials (statements by individuals that the treatment is working for them) and case studies. Although they may be suggestive, testimonials are the least reliable type of information. In fact, I have yet to find a treatment that does not have at least one proponent and one opponent. My attitude toward testimonials is this: If one person says something works well for them, I listen. If ten people say it works for them, I start doing some research to try to determine whether the substance has real value, or whether those ten people happened to get better due to other factors, while coincidentally taking the substance they claimed worked.

A more rigorous type of anecdotal evidence is the case study. Rather than just saying, for instance, that a person took SAMe and his joints felt better, a case study provides an in-depth analysis of an individual who received the treatment being researched. A case study starts with a physical description of the subject, including age, height, weight, and sex, as well as situations and life events that may be significant, such as occupation, stresses, traumas, relationships, family history, social situations, even beliefs and ideas. The case study goes on to describe in detail the patient's particular problem, such as osteoarthritis—which joints are affected, when they are affected and in what way, as well as any treatments that have already been tried and their results. Finally, it describes the treatment being tried, such as taking SAMe, and the results for this particular patient.

Case studies can be helpful for illuminating a particular disease-treatment process and the conditions surrounding it. Along with testimonials, they can suggest correlations that can then be investigated using more scientific methods. They have major disadvantages, however:

1. The sample size is very small, usually only one or a few persons.

2. There is no way to control for the influence of emotions and belief on the patient's condition.

The latter is known as the placebo effect. Belief is probably the most powerful healing tool humans have. It can probably even cure cancer. If we were strong enough and consistent enough to be able to work with the belief process, we probably wouldn't need medications at all. For most of us, however, emotions have a powerful, if erratic, effect on our health. Therefore, it can be extremely difficult to tell whether changes in a person's condition are the effects of a given treatment or the result of the person's belief that the treatment works.

Scientific Evidence

It is one thing to say that a treatment has apparently helped one person, ten people, or twenty people. To get a real sense of its effectiveness, however, we have to test it on large numbers of people, in the form of group studies. If we do the same thing with many different people and see the same or similar effects a significant amount of the time, we can begin to have confidence that a correlation actually exists between the treatment and the effects.

Group studies include three types: uncontrolled, single-blind, and double-blind. A fourth type, the meta-analysis or meta-study, combines multiple group studies to achieve an overall finding.

Uncontrolled Studies   In an uncontrolled study, everyone involved is aware of the treatment being given. In the case of SAMe, both the researchers and the subjects would know the subjects were taking SAMe. These studies may compare variations of the treatment, such as using different doses and time frames with different groups. If the studies show a positive correlation between the treatment and the desired effects, further testing may be necessary or appropriate.

The benefit of this kind of study is that you can use a number of different groups, and the cost is significantly lower than with more rigorous studies. The downside is that since both researchers and subjects know what is being used, their impressions and prejudices will certainly play a part. For example, people who believe in alternative medications may be much more amenable to believing that SAMe works and show subjective improvement as a result.

Single-Blind Studies   In a single-blind study, subjects are given either the test substance or a placebo. A placebo is an inert substance made into a form that closely resembles the substance being tested. The researcher knows what each subject is being given, but the subjects do not. This eliminates the emotional factor on the subject's side. However, it still leaves open the possibility that the researchers will unconsciously

niques used in the Commonwealth nations (particularly Canada, Australia, and South Africa) and in Europe are very similar to those used in the United States.

For most of us, . . . emotions have a powerful, if erratic, effect on our health. Therefore, it can be extremely difficult to tell whether changes in a person's condition are the effects of a given treatment or the result of the person's belief that the treatment works.

Like individuals, societies and cultures have intellectual and emotional biases that color not only how they interpret information, but what information they select to interpret in the first place. If we accept the existence of such biases, we can start to understand the distinctions between American researchers and those in other countries. For instance, researchers outside the United States are more likely to look critically on certain drugs and processes than researchers who come from the conventional American medical mold. It was Commonwealth studies, for example, that first demonstrated the weaknesses in the correlation between cholesterol levels and heart disease. Swedish studies first showed the dangers of thiazide diuretics almost two decades before those dangers were corroborated by American studies. Similarly, German studies are more apt to find benefits from herbs and homeopathics than American studies, because the German common bias favors the use of these preparations.

Rather than regarding such variations as differences in the quality of research, we need to take cultural biases into account and look at studies on a case-by-case basis. The fact that most of the studies of SAMe have been conducted in Europe reflects that continent's greater openness to options that are considered alternative in this country. It certainly does not make the results of those studies any less valid.

Analyzing Media Reports

Most lay people and even many doctors get most of their information about medical developments through media reports. These reports often quote from professional journals without noting that the information in the journal articles represents only a small piece of a giant puzzle that scientists are trying to solve.

An example is the recent coverage of a study examining the use of tamoxifen for preventing breast cancer. If you heard only the television news reports, you may have missed some of the study's most important findings, which were brought out in the journal article itself and some newspaper coverage. While the study indicated that approximately 50 percent of high risk women over 50 might avoid getting breast cancer by taking tamoxifen, it also indicated that those same women were at significant risk of getting blood clots in their legs (deep venous thrombosis), lungs (pulmonary embolism), or brains (strokes). A smaller number would get endometrial cancer. Nonetheless, the media hoopla over the study undoubtedly inspired numerous women to go to their doctors and demand that they be put on tamoxifen so that they will not get breast cancer.

The fact that most of the studies of SAMe have been conducted in Europe reflects that continent's greater openness to options that are considered alternative in this country. It certainly does not make the results of those studies any less valid.

The same kind of thing happened several years ago when women learned that they could find out whether they were at high risk for breast cancer by being tested for a certain gene. On discovering that they had the gene, a number of women opted for prophylactic mastectomies in order to prevent the onset of cancer. As bizarre as this draconian action may seem, some case might be made for it if there was a close correlation between the presence of the gene and the development of breast cancer. As it turned out, however, the correlation between having the gene and actually getting breast cancer is a poor one. The overwhelming majority of women who have the gene will never get breast cancer, and the overwhelming majority of women who do get breast cancer do not have the gene. This fact was known at the onset of the original study. Some years later, the association is finally being acknowledged as being too inconclusive to use as a basis for making medical decisions.

The best way to use media reports effectively is to let them bring issues to your awareness. If you become aware of a certain process or drug through the media, and it seems to have a reasonable relationship with your own health processes, then it may be worth investigating. You could do this by reading journals and medical databases. However, if you are not familiar with the language and process of medicine, you will have a difficult time interpreting what you read. A better approach is to talk with a caregiver whom you trust and who is knowledgeable not only about medical language and processes, but about your health and particular situation. A good caregiver should be willing to do some research in order to learn about new possibilities for treating her patients.

The Case for SAMe

So what does the scientific evidence suggest about SAMe? As we will see, based on a number of scientific, controlled studies, SAMe appears to have a positive effect on certain disease processes, including osteoarthritis, depression, and certain diseases of the liver. That is, taking SAMe affects these processes to the patient's benefit in a statistically significant number of cases. Out of a group of persons with osteoarthritis who take SAMe, a significant number will have less pain. At a molecular level, their joints will also show evidence of repair. Out of a group of persons with depression who take SAMe, a significant number will experience improved mood. The same is the case with cirrhosis of the liver.

. . . based on a number of scientific, controlled studies, SAMe appears to have a positive effect on certain disease processes, including osteoarthritis, depression, and certain diseases of the liver.

Thus, the evidence points to a pretty strong correlation between taking SAMe and experiencing improvements in any of these conditions. I'd like to say it is an exact cause-and-effect relationship, but if it were, every person who took SAMe would show improvement, and that's just not the case. Nor, however, is that the case with any medication available today. Just as the development of a disease depends on many factors, so too does the effectiveness of a given treatment. A person may respond positively to SAMe as a result of having a slightly better reparative processes than another person. Or SAMe might work better because the person's pain threshold is a little higher. There is just no way to determine in advance whether a given individual will fall into the majority who improve with SAMe or the minority who don't. I can say, however, that the odds are considerably better than any you would find in Las Vegas. At the very least, the risks are low, and the benefits for osteoarthritis, depression, and cirrhosis are sufficiently encouraging to make it worth trying.

CHAPTER 4

UNDERSTANDING OSTEOARTHRITIS

O f all the problems that SAMe may help, the evidence is strongest for its effects on osteoarthritis (OA), a painful and often debilitating condition that affects tens of millions of people. Current treatments for OA are limited to providing some symptomatic relief, and some of the treatments may actually do more harm than good, as we shall see. But SAMe appears not only to relieve arthritis pain, but to strengthen—and even rebuild—damaged cartilage. If this turns out to be true, many people would rightfully view SAMe as one of the most welcome medical discoveries in recent history. Before describing SAMe's potential benefits for arthritis sufferers, let's take a brief look at the disease itself, how it progresses, and how it is usually treated.

What Is Osteoarthritis?

The word "arthritis" is composed of the Greek word for joint, *arthron,* and the suffix *itis,* which means inflammatory disease or inflammation, hence, "inflammation of the joints." The term applies to a wide range of conditions that have the common characteristics of inflammation and pain in the joints. These include autoimmune diseases such as rheumatoid arthritis and lupus; gout, in which excess uric acid crystallizes in the joints; and a number of other relatively rare diseases. When most people speak of arthritis, however, they are referring to osteoarthritis (the prefix *osteo* means "bone"). This is an important distinction, because SAMe is helpful for OA, but not for any other form of arthritis. (Fibromyalgia, for which SAMe is also reportedly helpful, is technically not a form of arthritis at all, since it usually involves muscular rather than joint pain, and there is no detectable inflammation.)

OA is the third most common disease seen by family practitioners. It is slightly more common in women than men and increases in prevalence with age. A 45 year old has about a 2 percent chance of having OA, but for a 65 year old, the chance of having it jumps to 68 percent. The joints most commonly affected are those in the fingers, the thumb knuckle, knees, hips, low back, and neck, as well as the front of the shoulder, the base of the spine, and the jaw (the temporomandibular joint or TMJ).

What Causes Osteoarthritis?

Despite considerable research, we still don't know exactly what causes OA. Recent research indicates that the problem is a breakdown in the mechanism by which cartilage is produced and maintained, and that that breakdown actually occurs at a cellular level. (I'll talk more about this mechanism in Chapter 6.) We know that joint stress is a major factor in the development of OA, especially the stresses caused by obesity, repetitive motions, and major trauma such as sports injuries.

Obesity

Stress on a joint is like the physical stress on any structure. You could compare your skeleton and its joints to the framework of a bridge. A bridge that is kept in good repair and is not expected to support more weight than it was designed to carry will last a long time. But if a bridge is required to support more weight than it was designed for, the stress can damage or destroy it, even if it is well-built and maintained. Usually this does not happen all at once because of a single overload. Instead, the bridge is repeatedly stressed past its limits over a long period of time and gradually deteriorates.

When your joints are forced to carry more weight than they are meant to, the same thing happens to them. When a body is built to support 150 pounds, 200 pounds represents a 33 percent increase on that frame. In time, that increase will wear on the weight-bearing joints, namely the lumbar spine, sacroiliac joints, knees, and hips.

Mechanical Stress and Repetitive Motions

In addition to excess weight, joints can be stressed by repetitive motions and overuse. Joints that are used repetitively and with more stress are more likely to be affected. Thus, a seamstress or computer programmer is most likely to get OA in the fingers, while construction workers are more apt to get it in their hips and knees.

Major Trauma

Arthritis can also develop in joints that have been previously injured. Repeated injuries increase the likelihood of developing OA. Thus, certain high-injury sports are strongly implicated in OA. The worst of these is football, which repeatedly inflicts major trauma on various joints, particularly the shoulders, hips, and knees.

A Process of Degeneration

What happens in OA is a series of degenerative changes in the joint. First, the cartilage starts to break down at the areas of highest stress. At the same time, the bone underneath becomes harder, as if responding protectively to the stress, much like a callous forms on a farmer's hand. As the stress continues, the joint tries to repair itself in various ways. Cartilage shows evidence of self-repair. Bones around the joint develop spiny outgrowths called spurs. The joint lining (synovium) becomes inflamed, as the body attempts to remove and replace the damaged tissue. Blood vessels proliferate in an attempt to bring more healing to the area. Ultimately, the cartilage is worn down and bone rubs on bone. The effect is similar to what happens when brakes lose their lining and metal rubs against metal, except that the squeak is replaced by exclamations of pain!

As the joint damage progresses, more deformities can occur, all essentially as a result of the body's efforts to repair itself.

Cysts and nodes can form around the joint, especially in the fingers. The joint can make creaky or grating noises (crepitance) and fill with fluid. Joints can become unstable as they break down.

SAMe appears not only to relieve arthritis pain, but to strengthen—and even rebuild—damaged cartilage.

An OA-affected spine can present some special problems. The spinal vertebrae provide support and flexibility to the back and trunk, and serve as a bridge through which nerves travel from the neck to the arms and from the low back to the legs. When bone spurs form as part of the body's self-repair efforts, they can impinge on these nerves, causing pain, weakness, and numbness. This impingement is called radiculopathy. The area that is affected depends on which nerve is compromised. When radiculopathy occurs in the low back, it is also called sciatica, reflecting its impingement on a branch of the sciatic nerve. Surgery may be required to release the pressure on the affected nerve.

Symptoms and Effects

A person with an OA-affected joint feels an increasing limitation of movement, loss of dexterity, and increasing pain, usually described as a deep ache. At first the pain is relieved with rest, but as the deterioration continues, even rest provides no relief. Both stiffness and pain can be aggravated by weather changes, especially coldness and dampness—a big reason why Arizona is such a popular retirement destination. The stiffness is more pronounced when the joint has not been used for a period of time, such as when waking from sleep. Moving it improves the flexibility, as does heat. Arthritis-affected joints usually are not visibly inflamed—that is, they are not red or hot. There may be swelling, especially in the finger joints.

OA [osteoarthritis] is the third most common disease seen by family practitioners. It is slightly more common in women than men and increases in prevalence with age. A 45-year-old has about a 2 percent chance of having OA, but for a 65-year-old, the chance of having it jumps to 68 percent.

As any sufferer knows, OA can be debilitating. Only heart disease puts a greater limitation on a person's ability to perform daily functions. Eighty percent of people with OA have at least some limitations, and 25 percent are unable to perform at least one significant activity that is considered part of daily living. However, there are ways to mitigate the degenerative process. Probably the most important of these is movement. Moving an arthritic joint, as long as you take care not to overstress it, keeps it much more flexible. Even inflamed joints improve in function with movement.

Avoiding movement in an attempt to avoid pain actually leads to more stiffness, increased pain, and subsequently, greater limitation of motion. I have seen people who were barely able to move because their fear of pain was greater than their desire to be flexible. With help, however, many of them were able to overcome this problem, in large part due to their success in changing their attitudes about pain itself. Of course anything that helps to reduce the pain is welcome.

Distinguishing OA from Other Joint Conditions

In trying to determine whether the pain in a joint is caused by osteoarthritis or some other condition, we need to look past the joint itself to the structures that hold it together. A joint is more than a connection of two bones. It is a balanced system that includes:

- Bones for structure

- Ligaments to connect the bones

- Muscles to move the bones and keep them firm

- Tendons to connect the muscles to the bones

All of these components support one another, and a weakness in any component can cause problems throughout the system.

Strong muscles, for example, help reduce trauma to the joints and ligaments because they are better able to absorb the forces placed on the joints. If the muscles are weak, the tendons and ligaments must absorb some of the force. Sometimes they cannot handle the load, and they get injured. Joint pain more often indicates an injury to the tendon or ligament rather than to the joint itself. Any ligament or tendon can be injured. The most common injuries occur in the wrists (carpal tunnel syndrome), elbows (epicondylitis or tennis elbow), and knees (patellofemoral syndrome, also called chondromalacia or hamstring sprains). All of these injuries result from putting more force on a joint than it can withstand—either suddenly, as in a ski injury, or from repeated stresses over time, as in repetitive motion syndrome.

Tendon and ligament injuries are best treated with the following remedies:

- Ice

- Rest

- Support for the joint

- Anti-inflammatories

- Steroid injections (on occasion)

Gradually increasing strengthening exercises help in both healing and preventing further injury. SAMe does not help these kinds of conditions. This will be a significant observation when we look at the research on fibromyalgia, a nondegenerative condition characterized by chronic muscular pain.

The Value of Testing

Doctors have access to a whole array of tests, some of them very expensive, that we can use to learn more about the nature and severity of joint disorders. Unfortunately, the tests may not provide any additional information that would alter the course of treatment. A good clinician should be able to determine the nature and extent of OA with little testing. Some tests may be useful for distinguishing between the different types of arthritis, such as osteoarthritis and rheumatoid arthritis. If an examination suggests that a nerve is being compromised, tests can help determine the extent of nerve involvement.

A person with an OA-affected joint feels an increasing limitation of movement, loss of dexterity, and increasing pain, usually described as a deep ache.

Usually, however, the most rigorous—and most expensive—tests are also the most superfluous. Magnetic resonance imaging (MRI) is a good example of an overused diagnostic tool. Doing an MRI just because a patient has pain serves no purpose except possibly to reveal the extent of the damage. It will not provide any information that could help a doctor decide on a course of therapy. Why, then, are so many tests performed? Mainly because patients demand them. All too often, people insist on having X rays, CT scans, or MRIs without a clear understanding of what these tests are supposed to accomplish. I think this stems at least partly from the American reverence for technology, as well as from a misguided belief, or at least hope, that such state-of-the-art tests may somehow magically convey an aura of healing to the diseased area.

But MRIs and CT scans have neither healing nor diagnostic power; they are simply tools. Regardless of how much an MRI may detail, it is meaningless without a human being to interpret it. Likewise, a physician who uses only his eyes, and not his knowledge and intuition, is limited in his ability to diagnose, regardless of the quality of his tools. The art of medical diagnosis requires finely developed perceptions and a sense of knowing that goes beyond the capability of any technological marvel.

This is not to say that there aren't times when testing is useful. For example, an MRI may be appropriate if an examination reveals evidence of a nerve root compression like sciatica. In such cases the MRI can confirm the area and source of the compression, telling a surgeon whether surgery is truly necessary, and if so, exactly where to operate.

The Value of Tests for OA and RA

Many clinicians place a high value on radiography—that is, X rays. I am not so confident of their value with respect to OA. X rays are invaluable for determining the location and severity of broken bones. They are helpful, though not absolutely necessary, for finding pneumonia. The early stages of

OA, however, may not show up at all on X rays, while X rays at later stages may show great degeneration and damage. In my experience, there is no correlation between X ray findings and a patient's condition. I have seen patients with hot, swollen, and obviously painful joints whose X rays looked completely normal. On the other hand, I have observed horribly deformed spines, with bone spurs, compressed vertebral bodies, and narrowed joints, on X rays taken for other purposes where the individuals show no obvious arthritis symptoms.

As any sufferer knows, OA can be debilitating. Only heart disease puts a greater limitation on a person's ability to perform daily functions.

Certain blood tests can be helpful in distinguishing between OA and rheumatoid arthritis (RA), a completely different disease that does not respond to SAMe. RA is a systemic disease that affects the whole body, whereas OA attacks specific joints and affects only those joints. Tests such as sedimentation rate (ESR) and rheumatoid factor (RF) will show positive results in RA but not OA. Conventional medicine uses the same treatments for the initial stages of both RA and OA: anti-inflammatories, heat, range of motion exercises, and other basically conservative approaches.

But as each disease progresses, the treatments become widely divergent. Differentiating between the two makes it possible to identify the most appropriate course of treatment.

My wife has RA, which I diagnosed many years ago when I was first beginning my medical practice. She showed me symmetrical swelling of her knuckles (a symptom not found in OA) and complained of hip and knee pain. I couldn't find any other symptoms. I checked her sedimentation rate and rheumatoid factor, both of which were positive.

Not wanting to miss anything and, in view of my inexperience, desiring an expert opinion, I consulted a rheumatologist who ordered myriad blood tests, looking for liver, kidney, autoimmune, endocrine, and infectious causes. He also took X rays of every joint in her body. Every X ray was normal, and all blood and urine tests were negative, except the sedimentation rate and rheumatoid factor, thus confirming my original diagnosis. The specialist started her on ibuprofen and added a spectrum of RA-effective drugs when her symptoms were slow to abate. The battery of tests did nothing to change the diagnosis and subsequent treatment of my wife's RA. She does very well with it, with a lot of exercise, rest, and an anti-inflammatory.

My wife's experience illustrates how exhaustive testing does not necessarily improve either diagnosis or outcome. The time when tests may be most useful is for monitoring during treatment. This is because many medications, including those commonly used to treat OA, can have harmful effects on the body, as we shall see in the next chapter.

CHAPTER 5

CONVENTIONAL TREATMENTS FOR OSTEOARTHRITIS

Modern western medicine can tout many wonderful accomplishments. For example, if you are injured in a car crash or get shot or stabbed, you have a much greater chance of surviving today than you would have had a few years ago—assuming that the injuries are not immediately fatal and that you get hurt fairly close to a major trauma center. You also have a better chance of beating certain kinds of cancer, such as acute childhood leukemias, and numerous infectious diseases. We can replace your failing heart with a transplanted healthy one, re-attach your severed finger or ear, or bolster your supply of insulin if you are a diabetic.

When it comes to chronic conditions like OA, however, medical progress is not nearly so impressive. In fact, our most notable achievement regarding osteoarthritis may be that we've vastly increased people's chances of surviving long enough to get it. Having said that, let's look at what weapons western medicine does offer against arthritis, including surgical procedures, drugs, and therapies. We'll also look at what arthritis sufferers can do to help themselves, mainly through lifestyle changes such as weight control and exercise.

Surgical Procedures

The two types of surgery used for treating OA are arthroscopy and joint replacement. A joint degenerated by OA has shaggy cartilage, which can produce pain and noise and limit movement, especially if some of it breaks off and floats around the joint. Arthroscopy is used to clear debris out of the joint and smooth the shaggy cartilage, potentially offering years of relief. However, with each arthroscopy the cartilage gets thinner, so it cannot be done too many times.

Many arthroscopies are done as outpatient procedures, using tiny microscopes, fiber-optic technology, television, and special surgical tools that are inserted into the joint through small puncture wounds. This not only saves patients the pain and scarring of long incisions, but means less trauma and joint inflammation, and thus faster healing.

A more drastic option is replacing a joint, with hip replacements being the most common. Replacement becomes necessary when a joint has degenerated to a point where the patient cannot get any relief from the pain and is unable to move the joint. Joint replacement technology has been a tremendous boon to arthritis sufferers. Stories of successful joint replacements, especially in athletes of all ages, are numerous. Octogenarians have been able to return to playing tennis after hip replacement surgery. Joint replacement, however, is neither a cure nor a permanent solution for osteoarthritis. Artificial joints wear out more rapidly than natural ones, and the average life expectancy for major joints (such as hips and knees) is ten to fifteen years. So the odds are high that the replacement itself will eventually have to be replaced, perhaps several times.

With either arthroscopy or joint replacement, surgery alone is not enough to ensure relief from pain and stiffness, nor does it stop the degenerative process. With both types of treatment, a patient's overall health and fitness have a major impact on whether the surgery is successful and how long the effects last. In the case of arthroscopy, having and keeping strong muscles reduces the need for repeat procedures. The key to a solid recovery after a joint replacement is dedication to an intensive rehabilitation process. In a word, *movement* is essential to waging a successful battle against osteoarthritis at every stage, regardless of what other therapies are used.

Drug Treatments

The bad news is that relatively few drugs have any beneficial effect on osteoarthritis. By contrast, rheumatoid arthritis responds in varying degrees to a wide array of drugs that were originally used for other conditions. These include:

• Hydrochloroquine, for malaria

• Penicillinamine, for Wilson's disease (a liver ailment caused by excess copper)

• Sulfasalazine, used to treat inflammatory bowel disease

- Immunosuppressives, such as methotrexate, azathioprine, cyclophosphamide, and cyclosporin A, all of which have been used in various forms of cancer and to suppress immune responses in transplant patients

RA can also be helped by either oral doses or injections of gold (which is said by some to cure all ills). Lest you start to envy people with RA, however, you should realize that the effectiveness of these drugs is a decidedly mixed blessing, because they all come with a slew of side effects and organ toxicities.

. . . our most notable achievement regarding osteoarthritis may be that we've vastly increased people's chances of surviving long enough to get it.

For both RA and OA, the primary drug treatments consist of mild analgesics, or pain relievers, and nonsteroidal anti-inflammatory drugs, commonly called NSAIDs (pronounced en-sayds) or anti-inflammatories. For OA, these are effectively the *only* drug treatments. Unfortunately, they do nothing to retard the progress of the disease; at best they merely mask its symptoms.

Analgesics

The primary analgesics used to relieve arthritis pain are aspirin and acetaminophen. Aspirin is a very old and poorly understood drug whose many benefits we are only now starting to appreciate. The ancient Greeks used salicylic acid, a bitter powder derived from the bark of the willow tree, to relieve pain. In the late 1800s, a German industrial chemist named Felix Hoffman developed the first synthetic form of salicylic acid from coal tar. His employer, Bayer and Company, began marketing the product, acetyl-salicylic acid, under the name "aspirin" in 1897. The first known use of aspirin for treating arthritis was in 1899, when a medical colleague of Hoffman's named Heinrich Dreser used it to treat Hoffman's father, who suffered from RA.

Nobody is quite sure how aspirin works to relieve pain and inflammation, although there are many theories. We know that aspirin inhibits the synthesis and release of prostaglandins, which are hormones involved in a number of bodily processes. One type of prostaglandin that is produced in response to inflammation (such as in arthritic joints) may cause pain by increasing the sensitivity of pain receptors, the nerve endings that sense pain. Thus, decreasing prostaglandin production can also decrease pain. Additionally, aspirin may exert an analgesic effect on the hypothalamus, a part of the brain that is involved in how we *perceive* pain.

In addition to aspirin, other salicylates may be effective including salsalate and choline magnesium trisalicylate. These act similarly to aspirin and have similar side effects. All of the salicylates can cause gastrointestinal (GI) pain and bleeding if taken too frequently. They interfere with platelet function and may cause problems when combined with other drugs, notably warfarin (Coumadin). High doses can cause ringing in the ears, or tinnitus. In rare cases the liver or kidneys can be affected.

Some consider acetaminophen (the best known brand is Tylenol) to be the drug of choice for OA. It doesn't have the GI side effects of salicylates, but it also doesn't reduce inflammation the way aspirin does. This may not be that much of a drawback. Research in the past decade suggests that the anti-inflammatory effect is not as important as relieving pain, and acetaminophen does this quite well. Its major risk is the possibility of significant liver damage in toxic or high chronic doses.

NSAIDs

Like aspirin, NSAIDs have both analgesic and anti-inflammatory effects, and appear to work by inhibiting the synthesis and release of prostaglandins. The same prostaglandin-inhibiting activity makes NSAIDs, especially ibuprofen, effective against menstrual cramps. (One type of prostaglandin stimulates uterine contractions.)

NSAIDs come in several families based on their molecular configuration. At one time, researchers thought that these familial differences might offer varying benefits for different patients. This doesn't seem to be the case. In fact, neither I nor any doctor I have talked to has found any objective indicator that would help us direct patients to the correct NSAIDs for them. The latest variations are more likely the result of industry attempts to gain market share than discoveries that promise any new benefits to arthritis sufferers.

The most common NSAIDs used today are as follows (brand names are in parentheses):

- Indomethacin (Indocin)

- Ibuprofen (Advil, Motrin)

- Naproxen (Naprosyn)

- Toletin (Tolectin)

- Fenoprofen (Nalfon)

- Meclofenamate (Meclomen)

- Sulindac (Clinoril)

- Piroxicam (Feldene)

- Oxaprozin

- Diclofenac (Voltaren)

- Ketoprofen (Orudis)

- Nabumetone

- Etodolac

The proliferation of NSAIDs really began in the mid-seventies, with ibuprofen (best known under the brand names Motrin and Advil), which was followed by numerous others. Some of these are still on the market, while others have succumbed to the competition of the marketplace or the FDA's watchful eye. With each new discovery came the hope that it would be "the one." Butazolidine (Alka) showed promise for a time, but proved too toxic. Indomethacin was introduced in the early sixties and is still around today, despite a greater propensity than other NSAIDs to cause gastric irritation and bleeding.

Side Effects and Toxicity of Analgesics and NSAIDs

All of the medications I've discussed so far, regardless of their family name, dosages, and effectiveness, have common adverse effects that limit their use. Some people must add other medications in order to counteract the side effects. Sometimes the need to take other more crucial medications, such as blood thinners, will prevent a patient from using these drugs at all.

For both RA and OA, the primary drug treatments consist of mild analgesics, or pain relievers, and non-steroidal anti-inflammatory drugs, commonly called NSAIDS . . . or anti-inflammatories.

Gastrointestinal Problems   The most common adverse effect of both NSAIDs and aspirin is abdominal pain caused by irritation to the stomach lining. This can range from mild irritation causing transient pain to severe irritation causing gastritis, bleeding, and ulceration. The irritation may be dose-related, as in the patient who had blood in her stool only when she exceeded the recommended dose of the NSAID meclofenamate. Sometimes any dose is enough to cause problems, as in another patient who took the recommended doses of meclofenamate at two separate times and had heavy gastrointestinal (GI) bleeding each time, but no GI problems outside of these incidents.

Often, people take more than the recommended dosage and get away with it. All too often, however, even the recommended levels cause irritation. Taking the drugs with meals may help, but many patients require other medications to combat gastritis and reflux. The simplest solution, and often all that is needed, is an antacid. You can buy over-the-counter (OTC) stomach preparations that are exactly the same as what you would get with a prescription, only in smaller doses per tablet. For example, Tagamet is sold over the counter as 200 mg pills, while prescription Tagamet pills are 400 mg.

Ultimately, if the pain persists, or if bleeding cannot be controlled, it may be necessary to stop NSAIDs altogether. Switching to a different type of NSAID may help. In my experience, patients seem to have fewer GI problems with sulindac than with other NSAIDs, but this is only an anecdotal observation.

Blood Thinning   Due to their anti-prostaglandin activity, aspirin and NSAIDs interfere with platelet function and the blood's ability to clot. This blood-thinning effect has prompted the recent highly publicized claims that taking half an aspirin a day can lower the risk of heart disease. However, these drugs can cause internal bleeding when combined with other drugs that interfere with the clotting mechanism. The most notable of these is warfarin (Coumadin), which millions of Americans take in an effort to prevent heart attacks and strokes. Obviously, persons on warfarin cannot risk taking aspirin or NSAIDs. We used to think that they could take acetaminophen instead, but recent research indicates that combining acetaminophen with warfarin can also cause internal bleeding.

Kidney and Liver Damage Both NSAIDs and aspirin can cause kidney (renal) damage, although with aspirin this is rare. Prior to the advent of NSAIDs, a drug combination called APC (aspirin, phenacitin, and caffeine) was popular with headache sufferers. Phenacitin was widely known in medical circles to cause significant renal damage. Its popularity, in part, helped stimulate the search for an effective but less damaging medication. Although not as toxic as phenacitin, NSAIDs can contribute to a decreased flow of blood to the kidneys and resulting damage leading to fluid retention, loss of protein in the urine, high blood pressure, and renal failure. This risk is especially significant in people who may be prone to kidney damage, particularly diabetics.

Liver problems are also rare with both aspirin and NSAIDs, but hepatitis can occur with either. In addition, chronic use of NSAIDs can contribute to mild liver dysfunction. Acetaminophen, which is actually free of many of the side effects that plague the other analgesics, can be very toxic to the liver. Either chronic regular use or a single overdose can damage the liver so severely that a person can die from it. Acetaminophen poisoning is a medical emergency requiring attention in the intensive care unit. Alcohol use increases the liver toxicity of any of these drugs. If you consume more than two or three alcoholic drinks a day, you need to be aware of the potential for damaging your liver by combining alcohol and acetaminophen, aspirin, or NSAIDs.

Cartilage Destruction Ironically, both aspirin and NSAIDs may aggravate the very problems we are using them to treat. Recent research indicates that these drugs, along with steroids, may actually have properties that worsen the joint degeneration process. I'll discuss this more in the next chapter, when we compare conventional drug treatments with SAMe.

Other Effects   Both NSAIDs and aspirin can cause tinnitus (ringing in the ears), but aspirin is more likely to do so. In fact, physicians once used tinnitus as an indicator of the maximum dose a person could tolerate, and from there recommend a slightly lower dosage.

Other side effects found with NSAIDs are confusion, dizziness, anxiety, and drowsiness. However, these are common symptoms, especially in this high stress era. The best way to determine whether a particular symptom is related to the NSAID or has some other cause is to discontinue the medication for awhile and see if the symptom goes away.

Steroids

If a single joint is badly inflamed and swollen, a physician may inject it with a steroid such as cortisone. This is rarely a desirable option, however, as frequent steroid injections lead to less responsiveness and more degeneration, in addition to having other undesirable effects. Interestingly, steroids, in the form of ACTH, were once hailed as the magic bullet for arthritis, just as penicillin was supposed to be for streptococcal infections. When injected with ACTH, patients severely crippled with arthritis were dancing in the clinic. Unfortunately, the celebration was short-lived. The long-term side effects, which mimicked a disease of the adrenal cortex called Cushing's Disease, canceled out the short-term gains. Nevertheless, some physicians prescribe steroids, including oral drugs such as prednisone, for OA. Given the potential of steroids to harm people,

I believe this is an example of the treatment being worse than the disease.

Which Drug Is Best?

The truth is that no drug available in the United States has yet been demonstrated to be markedly better than aspirin for treating OA. Unfortunately, many patients, and not a few doctors, find it hard to believe that such a common and inexpensive drug can really be that effective, or else they are lured by the false assumption that newer is better. One thing is certain: Newer is more expensive, and aspirin is easily affordable, even the brand name varieties.

The best way to determine whether a particular symptom is related to the NSAID or has some other cause is to discontinue the medication for awhile and see if the symptom goes away.

In my experience, conventional treatment choices generally come down to an issue of cost versus how effective the patient *perceives* a drug to be. Because of the public's growing exposure to and awareness of medical options, many people have come to regard their doctors as obstacles to whatever treatment the patient already believes to be appropriate rather than as professionals whose expertise can support the patient's well-being. This attitude leads to a tendency to deride over-the-counter (OTC) preparations as being less effective than the prescription variety. Similarly, many people believe that generic drugs are less potent than the brand name versions. But I'm going to let you in on a well-kept secret of the pharmaceutical industry: Despite Madison Avenue's apparently successful efforts to convince us otherwise, the vast majority of generics are just as good as their brand name counterparts. This includes OTC analgesics such as aspirin, ibuprofen, and acetaminophen.

I can't tell you how often patients come to me asking for relief from arthritis pain, having already tried OTC's without success. They insist on a prescription for what amounts to the *exact same thing* they're already taking! For example, a patient who gets no relief by taking three 200-mg tablets of Advil four times a day goes home with a prescription for 600-mg tablets of ibuprofen to be taken four times a day, and reports back that it worked. No amount of logic can convince these patients that the medicine and the doses are the same. Alternatively, one person will not feel any effect from one brand of ibuprofen, but do well on another.

If these reports came down consistently against a particular medication, I would infer that the drug itself was deficient, but no such pattern has ever revealed itself. The same paradox occurs when it comes to varieties of NSAIDs. One patient may not get relief with ibuprofen, but do well with naproxen. Both of these belong to the same family of NSAIDs, the propionic acid derivatives. Recently, I switched one patient from ibuprofen to diclofenac and another from diclofenac to ibuprofen. Both experienced relief.

Therefore, my approach to arthritis treatment has been largely cost-driven. I start with the least expensive alternatives first and work my way up. This means that patients who do not find relief until trying the more costly NSAID may suffer a while longer than they would otherwise. But since I don't have any assurance that the most expensive medications are also the most effective, I may as well start by identifying the patients who will do best on ibuprofen or aspirin. When it comes to SAMe, however, it's possible that cost considerations will take a back seat to safety and effectiveness.

Therapies

The main objective in arthritis therapy is to keep the affected joints strong and flexible—to keep them moving, but not in a way that could cause more damage or trauma. One way to do this is by manipulation, either chiropractic or osteopathic. Manipulation helps reduce the muscle tension that is the result of the pain and the stiffness the muscles have to move against. It also directly increases the mobility of the joint. Another way of improving mobility and reducing muscle tension is massage therapy. Massage helps keep the muscles more relaxed by removing any spasms around the joint. Both types of therapy also help patients experience the range of motion that is possible with their affected joints. Soaking in hot water can also be very helpful, such as in a sitz bath, jacuzzi, or hot tub. In fact, any type of heat is very beneficial for stiff, arthritic joints. Using all these therapies in combination is also an effective treatment for mild to moderate injuries or joint stresses—both for relieving the immediate pain and for helping to prevent the onset of major degeneration.

A device that has been around for about two decades is a low level electrical stimulation unit called TENS (transcutaneous electrical nerve stimulation). Many people have found a TENS unit to be effective for localized chronic pain. When it works, TENS is a godsend. It probably is not used as much as it could be.

In a word, movement *is essential to waging a successful battle against osteoarthritis at every stage, regardless of what other therapies are used.*

Acupuncture also could be effective for OA. If you decide to try acupuncture, be sure you go to someone who has graduated from an accredited school of Chinese medicine and who is knowledgeable in all aspects of the "five element" theory. People who have learned acupuncture from less than a complete program may not have the skills needed to perform acupuncture effectively.

Some people claim that magnets are effective for relieving the pain of arthritis and other conditions. I don't find this type of treatment effective. It is expensive and of dubious benefit.

Lifestyle Approaches

Virtually all OA can be attributed to stresses on the joints caused by obesity, mechanical stress, repetitive motion, and/or trauma. Once the degenerative process has started, any of these stresses will aggravate the deterioration of a joint. Thus, controlling your weight, avoiding overstressing joints, and keeping your muscles strong and flexible can help prevent arthritis from occurring in the first place or slow its progress once it does occur. This is not something any doctor, therapist, pill, or injection can do for you. You must do it for yourself.

Weight Control

As I pointed out in the last chapter, the more excess weight you are carrying around, the more stress you are putting on your joints. It is generally accepted that joints can tolerate a 20 percent increase over what is considered ideal weight. Thus, maintaining your weight within that range is a good way to prevent or slow the progress of OA. A good rule of thumb for determining your appropriate height to weight ratio is as follows:

- If you are a woman, start with a baseline of 100 pounds, and add five pounds for every inch over five feet. Thus, if you are 5'4", your ideal weight is 120 pounds. The maximum acceptable weight is 20 percent more, or 144 pounds.

- If you are a man, start with a baseline of 106 pounds, and add six pounds for every inch over five feet. This means if you are 5'9", your ideal weight is 160 pounds. When the 20 percent is added, the maximum acceptable weight is 192 pounds.

Establishing a good weight control program is well outside the scope of this book, but there is a lot of help available should you choose to seek it out. There is no avoiding the basic formula, however. It consists of two simple things: eat less and move more.

In my experience, conventional treatment choices generally come down to an issue of cost versus how effective the patient perceives a drug to be.

Avoiding Mechanical Stress

The best way to counteract the stress of repetitive movements and heavy mechanical stressors is a combination of rest and strengthening exercises. Unfortunately, most people continue to do activities that make their joints hurt without trying to make them stronger. John Elway is still at the top of his form, after 15 years in the National Football League, in large part due to his rigorous training schedule both on- and off-season. This strengthening has compensated for numerous injuries and surgeries. It is unlikely, however, despite the training, that he will escape some long-term joint pains and OA. Even the best-conditioned NFL athletes suffer this consequence. Dick Butkus has discussed the daily pain that he endures as a result of his NFL experience. It's a similar story for a data entry clerk with OA in her hands and fingers, or a construction worker whose spine shows the effects of repeatedly lifting 150-pound loads of Sheetrock every day for many years.

Even after the degeneration of OA has begun, range of motion exercises, muscle strengthening exercises, and activities to increase the joint's endurance will decrease pain and increase function. Biomechanics, which involves analyzing the ways people hold and move their bodies, can also be helpful for identifying and correcting patterns that may be causing additional stress to the joints.

For those with serious OA, supportive devices like canes, crutches, and walkers reduce the chance of maladaptive walking behaviors that can increase stress on the diseased joint or its opposite counterpart. It's not uncommon, for example, to develop pain in your good knee as a result of favoring the OA-affected knee. There are many helpful gadgets and devices that can make life with OA easier, such as jar openers, pen and pencil grips, Velcro fasteners, and even special key rings with levers to help you turn a key in an ignition or door lock.

Exercise—Move It or Lose It

Although rest is recommended for short periods of time, the worst thing you can do for OA is to stop moving. Lack of activity will cause the affected joint to freeze and lead to even greater pain when it is used. Many people who have been sedentary for years get into a disastrous cycle of trying to reduce pain by reducing activity, which leads to more pain and even less activity, which results in a vicious cycle. Exercise is important not only for weight control but for strengthening muscles and maintaining flexibility, which in turn reduces stress on the joints. It also makes you feel better!

. . . controlling your weight, avoiding overstressing joints, and keeping your muscles strong and flexible can help prevent arthritis from occurring in the first place or slow its progress once it does occur.

This doesn't mean you should sign up at a gym and start a concentrated fitness program. What it means is that you should move whenever possible. It's particularly important to do exercises that build up the muscles around the joint—the stronger the muscles, the more stable the joint, and the less damage can occur to it. Walking is, of course, the simplest exercise. It takes no special equipment, other than a good pair of shoes, and can be done almost anywhere. If walking is too difficult or painful, swimming and water walking are very beneficial activities that require nothing more than access to a warm swimming pool. Many recreation centers have inexpensive water exercise programs specifically geared for people with arthritis.

Any exercise program should include stretching exercises to keep muscles flexible and avoid injury. Yoga, which involves gentle stretches, is excellent for improving both flexibility and strength in all the muscle groups and joints. Done in a peaceful setting and with a focused attitude, it also fosters relaxation and proper breathing, and can be used to achieve a quiet, almost meditative state. The slow, patterned movements of tai chi are also excellent for improving circulation, range of motion, and balance, as well as promoting relaxation and focused attention.

All in all, exercise, weight control, and simple remedies like soaking in a hot bath may be the best weapons you have against arthritis. At least they do not carry the side effects and potential for harm that the commonly used drugs do. Still, many OA sufferers can't help feeling that they ought to have some better options. As we shall see, they do—and SAMe is at the top of the list.

SAMe AND OSTEOARTHRITIS

As I explained in the previous chapter, conventional western medicine does not have much to offer in the way of ammunition against osteoarthritis. All of the drugs currently used to treat OA provide only symptomatic relief, if that, while doing nothing to retard the progress of the disease. They carry a heavy risk of side effects and potential for organ damage. And as a supreme irony, they actually appear to contribute to cartilage destruction, thus worsening the condition they are supposed to alleviate. Further, while lifestyle changes such as weight control and exercise can help slow the progress of the disease, they cannot reverse the damage that has already been done.

It is possible, however, that SAMe offers an alternative that is not only much safer and less toxic than conventional drugs, but that actually helps to rebuild damaged cartilage and stop the degenerative process of OA. Let's look at just what that possibility entails.

Understanding the Joints

In order to understand how SAMe works to counteract OA, it helps to know a little about joints and the mechanisms by which cartilage is produced, maintained, and destroyed. At the base of a joint are the bones themselves. On top of and lining the bones where they connect is a layer of cartilage. Surrounding the cartilage, at the border of cartilage and bone, is a firm lining of connective tissue called synovium. Thus the joint, bordered by synovium, is fairly self-contained.

The cartilage itself is a complex mechanism that has three main components. One component consists of cells called chondrocytes, which are the only living tissue in the joint. As part of the manufacturing process, the chondrocytes make chondroitin sulfate, a substance that is used to make the molecules that go into cartilage and other soft connective tissue such as ligaments, tendons, and bone. Chondroitin sulfate is also a precursor to glucosamine, which I'll talk about a little later in the chapter. The other components of the cartilage are collagen and proteoglycan, both of which are manufactured by the chondrocytes. Collagen is a highly stable matrix, or network, of connective tissue. It is somewhat firm, but can become brittle if struck directly, rather like a piece of hard rubber. The proteoglycan, which is much less stable, lines the outside of the collagen. One of the functions of the proteoglycan is to hold water, which, in conjunction with the collagen, serves as a cushion in the cartilage.

Proteoglycan production is a dynamic process. The proteoglycan is constantly breaking down and being built up. In healthy individuals, this process is balanced: As much new proteoglycan is being made as is being destroyed.[1] This is similar to what goes on in other high-production, high-wear organs of the body, such as the skin. Epithelial (skin) cells are constantly dying as a natural process of wear and tear on the skin. They also die as a result of trauma, temperature extremes, or dryness. You might think that the constant loss of cells would cause considerable damage to the skin, which would become thinner and finally break down. That doesn't happen, however, because new cells are being made as fast as the old cells are dying.

It is possible . . . that SAMe offers an alternative that is not only much safer and less toxic than conventional drugs, but that actually helps to rebuild damaged cartilage and stop the degenerative processes of OA.

Placing physical stress on a joint contributes to the destruction of proteoglycan and collagen, while also inhibiting the ability of the chondrocytes to produce more of these substances.[2,3] The chondrocytes are embedded in and surrounded by the cartilage matrix. Unlike most other cells, which have a close connection to their food supply, the chondrocytes are so deeply embedded in the cartilage tissue that glucose must go through circuitous channels to reach them. Damage to the cartilage can reduce the availability of glucose to the chondrocytes, thus setting up a destructive feedback loop—the less energy the chondrocytes get, the less ability they have to repair the cartilage. Fortunately, however, chondrocytes are hardy cells that have an ability to live without glucose longer than other cells, keeping them viable for a long time. However, if the chondrocytes are unable to maintain normal production, or if a significant amount of the proteoglycan and collagen matrix (also called glycosaminoglycans) is destroyed and the chondrocytes aren't able to keep up with repairs, the joint will begin to break down.[4-6] In other words, osteoarthritis will develop. Thus, the key to preventing or slowing the process of osteoarthritis is keeping the existing matrix of collagen and proteoglycan strong and maintaining the ability of the chondrocytes to do their job.[7]

The Problem with Drugs

Evidence is mounting that virtually all the drugs currently used to treat OA, including salicylates (aspirin), NSAIDs, and steroids, have a destructive effect on cartilage.[8-11] The mechanisms of this destruction may be different for each type of drug. However, both NSAIDs and aspirin contribute to cartilage destruction by suppressing the ability of the chondrocytes to synthesize proteoglycan and inhibiting the enzymes that help to manufacture chondroitin sulfate.[12-16] The depletion of proteoglycan leaves the chondrocytes themselves much more vulnerable to damage.[17] A cascading effect occurs, starting with damaged cartilage.[18,19] The drugs enter the joint and inhibit the production of chondroitin or proteoglycan. This causes the chondrocytes to become embedded even more deeply in the matrix, thus further damaging their ability to produce proteoglycan. Interestingly, the anti-inflammatories are more destructive to damaged cartilage, as in osteoarthritis, than they are to normal cartilage. This appears to be because the damaged cartilage takes up the NSAIDs more readily than does normal cartilage.[20]

The realization that current treatments may be doing more harm than good has stimulated the search for a drug that is "chondroprotective," that is, that would reduce the pain and inflammation of OA without doing additional harm to the cartilage itself.

Evidence also shows that steroids, although they can reduce inflammation, inflict significant damage on the chondrocytes. This damage is even greater than that caused by some anti-inflammatories and results in an increased amount of dead chondrocyte cells. One study compared patients in a control group with patients receiving an NSAID (indomethacin), and patients receiving a steroid (dexamethazone). At the end of the study, the control group had 3.7 dead cells out of a hundred, the indomethacin group had 10.7 dead cells per hundred, and the dexamethazone group had 16.6 dead cells out of a hundred.[21]

The Search for Chondroprotective Agents

The realization that current treatments may be doing more harm than good has stimulated the search for a drug that is "chondroprotective"—that is, that would reduce the pain and inflammation of OA without doing additional harm to the cartilage itself. A number of substances show promise in this area, although their actual effectiveness is controversial. These substances include: diacerin, glucosamine,[22] a compound called CN-100,[23] and SAMe.

SAMe works by supporting greater production of proteoglycan. Since this is the high-wear, high-production component of cartilage, enhancing its production goes a long way toward protecting the rest of the cartilage matrix.

What the Research Shows About SAMe and OA

The clinical research on SAMe extends back two decades. Although the original research was done in Europe, later and more extensive research was conducted in the United States, although it has somehow escaped public notice. In fact, it's been a full decade since a review of the literature on SAMe appeared in the prestigious *American Journal of Medicine*.[24] The review examined studies involving a total of 22,000 patients.[25] These studies looked at SAMe's effectiveness on OA in comparison with NSAIDs and placebos, as well as its side effects and its effects on cartilage tissue. What they found has promising implications for OA sufferers.

Animal Studies

Though many people regard it as unnecessarily cruel, medical animal research has saved millions of human lives and reduced the suffering of countless others. For obvious reasons, we cannot subject humans to the kind of intensity and control that characterize animal studies. For example, we can't use an arthroscope to take samples of cartilage from human joints for testing. Even if it were ethically acceptable to do so, the process itself would contribute to the deterioration of the cartilage, thus negating any positive effects of the drug being tested.

Of course, it is up to each person to decide whether to support animal research. Those who choose not to do so, however, if their position is to have any integrity, would also need to refrain from using many of the products, drugs, medical procedures, and basic social conveniences that have come to us by way of animal testing. This would essentially preclude getting any modern medical attention, since virtually all medical research involves animals at one time or another. For many treatments, these studies are extensive and ongoing. Each rat, monkey, rabbit, or gerbil that succumbs in a laboratory has the potential to improve the quality and safety of our lives.

One alternative to blanket protests against all animal research is to support policies that keep it to a minimum. We need to recognize when sufficient research has been conducted in a given area, and prevent additional or repeat studies from being done unnecessarily. We can also identify and eliminate studies that are irrelevant or self-serving. Using animals is essential, but so is using them wisely and judiciously. Having said that, let's look at some of the animal research involving SAMe.

In one study, chickens were injected with a substance that caused their knee joints to degenerate. Each chicken received a weekly injection of SAMe into one knee joint, while the other joint served as the control; that is, it was left to follow its natural course of progressive degeneration as a result of the first injection of poison. At the end of the study, the chickens' knee joints were examined. The SAMe-injected joints showed significantly less deterioration than the untreated joints.[26]

The same study was conducted on rabbits, with similar results. After 12 weeks, the control joints showed much greater degeneration than the SAMe-treated joints, demonstrating SAMe's ability to protect the cartilage against degenerative elements. Furthermore, the cartilage of the animals who received SAMe injections showed a significant increase in proteoglycan, confirming that SAMe was actually contributing to the growth of cartilage.[27,28]

Human Studies

As I stated before, we cannot take human cartilage samples for study, especially from people who are already losing cartilage to disease. Therefore, human studies examine symptoms and signs. OA symptoms consist of participants' reported levels of pain under different conditions, such as rest, walking, climbing stairs, or swimming. Signs are objective findings, which are easier to measure. These include:

- Crepitation, the amount of noise a joint makes when being manipulated

- Swelling, as measured by the joint's circumference

- Mobility, or the extent of a joint's range of motion

- How fast the subject can walk ten meters

The largest study involved 20,641 patients who received SAMe for eight weeks. Seventy-one percent of the participants reported "good" or "very good" benefits, while only 9 percent reported poor outcomes. Eighty-seven percent tolerated the supplement very well. Five percent dropped out due to intolerance, and 2.3 percent dropped out due to lack of benefit.[29]

The longest study followed 108 patients for two years. Participants started at 200 mg three times a day, then went to a maintenance dose of 200 mg twice a day. No one discontinued therapy due to side effects, and no adverse effects were reported in the last six months of the study. The results were generally positive. Reported benefits included a significant decrease both in morning stiffness and in pain at rest and at motion. Significantly, patients who had been suffering from depression along with OA experienced relief from those symptoms as well—a finding that we will study more closely in Chapter 9.[30]

Comparing SAMe with Placebos and Existing Drugs

Different studies measured SAMe's effectiveness against various NSAIDs and placebos. The NSAIDs studied were naproxen, ibuprofen, indomethacin, and piroxicam.

Two studies compared SAMe and naproxen. One lasted for six weeks and involved 20 people;[31] the other lasted 28 days and involved 33 centers and 734 people.[32] For SAMe, the initial therapeutic dose was 400 mg three times a day, which was reduced to a maintenance dose of 400 mg twice a day. For naproxen, the initial dose was 250 mg three times a day and the maintenance dose was 250 mg twice a day. A third group of patients received a placebo. SAMe was as effective as the naproxen; patients on both drugs showed a marked improvement. The SAMe patients experienced less GI disturbance than those on naproxen. Interestingly, while 10 patients dropped out of the study due to side effects from SAMe, 13 dropped out due to side effects from the placebo.

Two studies, each lasting four weeks, were conducted comparing SAMe and ibuprofen, one involving 36 patients,[33] and one with 150 patients.[34] The studies showed no difference between the two drugs with respect to either beneficial or adverse effects. No one dropped out of these studies.

In summary, SAMe has received a fair trial in clinical studies, all of which demonstrated both its effectiveness and a much better side effect profile as compared to NSAIDs.

Two one-month studies compared SAMe with indomethacin; one involved 36 patients;[35] the other involved 90 patients.[36] Again there were no differences in beneficial effect. Two patients had slight transient nausea from taking SAMe. In the latter study, it was discovered that SAMe did not have any beneficial effect on rheumatoid arthritis. SAMe also compared favorably to piroxicam in an 84-day study.[37] Piroxicam showed significant benefits over a placebo alone in two other studies.[38, 39]

In summary, SAMe has received a fair trial in clinical studies, all of which demonstrated both its effectiveness and a much better side effect profile as compared to NSAIDs. Perhaps most important, SAMe apparently possesses the long-sought for chondroprotective benefits. In fact, it actually demonstrated an ability to foster cartilage growth, unlike the NSAIDs, which contribute to cartilage deterioration. And unlike NSAIDs and acetaminophen, it does not appear to hold any potential for kidney, liver, or other organ damage.

Why SAMe's Benefits Remain Unrecognized

Why hasn't SAMe been used extensively in the more than ten years since the publication of these studies in a well recognized, well refereed journal ("refereed" means the studies were examined by respected researchers before they were published)? Several possibilities come to mind. Some are relatively benign, reflecting habit and human nature rather than deliberate intent; others are more nefarious.

Doctors get their information about new drugs and treatment protocols primarily from two sources: medical journals and sales representatives from pharmaceutical companies. This is partly because keeping up with the latest in medical research and treatment protocols is an overwhelming task, and partly because, like everyone else, doctors have selective attention. It's a truism of popular advertising that information must be repeated several times before it takes root in someone's mind. The rule of thumb in television is that a viewer must see the same commercial six times before he remembers it (even then there is no guarantee he will remember, much less purchase, the product being advertised).

As consumers of medical information, doctors are no different from the audiences targeted by advertisers. A topic must be addressed in several medical journals over a relatively short period of time in order to get their attention. One or two articles here and there are not enough to do the trick. (The exception is when an article in the *Journal of the American Medical Association (JAMA)* or the *New England Journal of Medicine* gets picked up by the mass media, where it may catch the attention of patients/consumers and eventually trickle through to doctors. Obviously that did not happen with the SAMe literature review.) Additionally, just like publishers of popular magazines, publishers of medical journals are more likely to be trend followers than trend setters. Medical journals also naturally tend to reflect the conservatism of the profession itself, so alternative treatments get short shrift.

. . . unlike NSAIDs and acetaminophen, [SAMe] does not appear to hold any potential for kidney, liver, or other organ damage.

Another possibility for the lack of recognition of SAMe's benefits has to do with the tremendous influence of pharmaceutical companies on what treatments doctors prescribe and use. Doctors and pharmaceutical representatives have a relationship similar to that of members of Congress and lobbyists. Doctors rely on the representatives for most, if not all, of their information about what drugs are best for treating certain conditions, despite their recognition that the representatives are obviously biased sources of information. It has long been a concern both within the medical profession and the federal government that pharmaceutical companies may exert undue influence on doctors' treatment decisions, particularly as the pharmaceutical companies often "court" doctors with gifts, meals, and other perks. Supplements are not usually marketed as aggressively as pharmaceuticals. If SAMe were to come to the attention of a major pharmaceutical company that could produce it in a patented form, no doubt doctors and patients would hear about it. But then it would likely be available only as a prescription drug, with all the complications that that entails.

How Much SAMe Is Needed for OA?

Given existing information, recommending a specific dosage is difficult. The amounts used in the studies cited above ranged from 600 to 1,600 mg a day. In his book, *Encyclopedia of Nutritional Supplements,* Dr. Michael Murray suggests an initial dose of 200 mg twice a day (400 mg/day), increasing to 400 mg three times a day (1,200 mg/day), then eventually dropping back to a maintenance dose of 400 mg a day.[40]

The issue of dosage becomes important when cost is taken into consideration, as the long-term cost of taking 1,600, or even 1,200 mg, of SAMe a day would be prohibitive for most people, given SAMe's current price levels. Hopefully, more research over the next few years will help us arrive at a realistic (and affordable) dosage. In the meantime, the best recommendation I can give is to let your symptoms be your guide. Take more when your symptoms are worse, and less when you are feeling better. Additionally, since SAMe will not work if a person has low levels of B12 and folate, you should also take these supplements while taking SAMe. A dosage of one mg each per day is sufficient.

Oral versus Intramuscular or Intravenous SAMe

A number of the studies cited involved intramuscular or intravenous administration of SAMe. This may be because an oral form was not available until fairly recently. In any case, most people do not have daily access to someone who can administer such injections, and even if they did, they would probably prefer to take SAMe orally. The evidence suggests that oral administration is effective for OA. I'll discuss this more in Chapter 14.

Other Alternative Treatments for OA

You can find many alternative treatments for arthritis at your local health food store—or possibly even in your spice rack or backyard. You have probably heard of the book *The Arthritis Cure,* which extols the virtues of glucosamine sulfate and chondroitin sulfate for treating arthritis. We'll take a brief look at herbal remedies, then see how the more well-known supplements stack up to SAMe.

Herbs

Among the herbs that are touted as helpful for arthritis are devil's claw, curicumin, and feverfew, all of which are alleged to have anti-inflammatory properties. Other natural anti-inflammatories include white oak bark, white willow bark (a good substitute for aspirin), and plantain leaves.

Devil's Claw The scientific name for devil's claw is *Harpogophytum procumbens.* It is a tuber, or root, found in southern and eastern Africa. Studies in France and Germany have compared the anti-inflammatory action of devil's claw to that of the steroids cortisone and phenylbutisone. The recommended dosage is ¼ to ½ teaspoon of the extract three times a day.

Devil's claw is often used in conjunction with other herbs. One of these is *menyanthes apium,* or celery seed, which is indigenous to England and is also found in Europe and North America. Apium is also good for gout and inflammation of the urinary tract, and appears to have some anti-depressive effects.

. . . since SAMe will not work if a person has low levels of B12 and folate, you should also take these supplements while taking SAMe. A dosage of one mg each per day is sufficient.

Another herb used with devil's claw is *Gaultheria,* or wintergreen. Gaultheria is an evergreen shrub found throughout the eastern United States and Canada, from which comes methyl salicylate, which we also know as a form of aspirin (acetyl salicylic acid). *Dioscorea villosa,* also called wild yam root or colic root, can also be used in combination with devil's claw. It is also found in the eastern and central United States and has been shown to be beneficial, not only as an anti-inflammatory, but also as an anti-spasmodic. It's of particular benefit in the acute phase of rheumatoid arthritis, and is sometimes referred to as "rheumatism root."

Pregnant women should not take devil's claw.

Curicumin   *Curicuma longa,* also called turmeric, is purported to be a powerful anti-inflammatory, as well as having numerous other properties. The recommended dosage is ¼ to 1 teaspoon of the extract three times a day.

Feverfew   Feverfew, also called *Tanacetum parthenium,* is credited with a host of beneficial effects, including working as an anticoagulant, anti-inflammatory, anti-microbial, anti-pyretic, anti-spasmodic, digestive, expectorant, vasodilator, and stimulant. Its traditional uses include treatment of arthritis, asthma, colic, colitis, the common cold, depression, diarrhea, headache, ear ache, fever, indigestion, insomnia, intestinal worms, liver disorders, migraine, nausea, rheumatism, stomach ache, and vomiting. For arthritis, the recommended dose is 1 to 2 tablets three times a day, or ¼ to 1 teaspoon of the extract three times a day, with juice or water.

Glucosamine Sulfate

To understand how this supplement might work, let's go back to our description of a joint. Remember that the main constituents of joint cartilage are the chondrocytes, collagen, and proteoglycan. Glucosamine supports the build-up of proteoglycan, and seems to do so in a dose-dependent way. This is where it is the most beneficial, rather than as a pain reliever. However, even though it is not an analgesic as such, it actually does provide significant pain relief in affected joints.

Considering the evidence, I would recommend the supplements over any of the traditional drugs, with SAMe demonstrating more overall effectiveness at this point than either glucosamine or chondroitin.

Because the section of the proteoglycan that most needs building up includes a sulfated portion, glucosamine sulfate has been demonstrated to be the most effective and appropriate form. In fact, various experiments have demonstrated that compared to other forms of glucosamine such as N-acetylglucosamine or glucosamine hydrochloride, glucosamine sulfate is clearly superior in absorption.

Studies have shown that supplementation with glucosamine increases the amounts of both glycosaminoglycans and chondroitin sulfate in the areas of the cartilage that are being repaired. This suggests that these substances are important in the repair of damaged cartilage.[41-45] People with both rheumatoid arthritis and osteoarthritis also have increased amounts of glucosamine in their urine—which may actually make glucosamine a good marker for active cases of arthritis. Also, both chondroitin and glucosamine seem to decrease with age, suggesting that joint degeneration in older adults may be at least in part due to the decreased availability of these building blocks for repairing cartilage tissue.[46,47]

As far as clinical effectiveness, glucosamine seems to work quite well, although not as well as SAMe. One study matched it against ibuprofen in 40 patients over an eight-week period.[48] The patients received either 500 mg of glucosamine three times a day (TID), or 600 mg of ibuprofen two times a day (BID). Although the pain decreased more rapidly in the ibuprofen group, the patients receiving glucosamine demonstrated a more enduring decrease in pain, going up to the eighth week. In another study, patients received 400 mg of glucosamine sulfate (GS) intramuscularly for the first seven days. They were then divided into two groups. Patients in one group received a maintenance dose of 1,500 mg of GS each day for two weeks, while the other group received a placebo. All subjects showed marked improvement in the first week. The GS group demonstrated continued improvement on the maintenance dose, whereas the placebo group went back to the original level of pain.[49]

In another experiment, 155 outpatients received IM injections of either 400 mg of glucosamine sulfate or a placebo twice a week for six weeks. Again, there was a significant decrease in pain and increase in mobility in the glucosamine-treated subjects.[50]

Dosage and Side Effects   The accepted dosage for glucosamine sulfate is 500 mg three times a day. Alternatively it can be given as 400 mg IM injections two to four times a day, although this is obviously less appropriate.

Few side effects are associated with glucosamine sulfate, as it is a substance that is naturally made in the body. The only reported effects are mild gastrointestinal problems (indigestion, diarrhea, nausea, or heartburn), which can generally be avoided by taking it with food.

Chondroitin Sulfate

Less information is available regarding the efficacy of chondroitin sulfate for osteoarthritis. Chondroitin sulfate, you'll recall, is one of the substances made by the chondrocytes. It is an important component of the proteoglycan, particularly with respect to its ability to catch and hold water in the cartilage matrix, a process that seems to involve the chondroitin sulfate attaching to the glucosamine. This has led some people to believe that adding chondroitin sulfate to the glucosamine sulfate enhances the ability of both substances to repair the cartilage tissue. Some also recommend using gelatin for the same reason.

Although the theory seems to have some merit, there have not been enough studies to demonstrate whether this is truly the case. If you decide to take chondroitin sulfate, however, the recommended dose is 400 mg three times a day. A number of glucosamine-chondroitin combination preparations are available, some of which also include gelatin. Persons who weigh more than 200 pounds should increase the dose somewhat for both substances.[51]

All three substances—glucosamine sulfate, chondroitin sulfate, and SAMe—are chondroprotective agents, and are therefore more likely to benefit arthritis sufferers than the anti-inflammatories. Considering the evidence, I would recommend the supplements over any of the traditional drugs, with SAMe demonstrating more overall effectiveness at this point than either glucosamine or chondroitin. It is certainly worth trying for at least 60 days to see if you gain any benefits.

CHAPTER 7

UNDERSTANDING DEPRESSION

Depression is one of the most enigmatic diseases of the late twentieth century. It is also one of the most common—an estimated 3 to 5 percent of Americans are diagnosed with it each year. Older people are more likely to be depressed than younger ones; more than 50 percent of adults between 60 and 70 years of age who are hospitalized for any reason are also depressed. These numbers do not include those who are diagnosed with other illnesses in which depression may be a factor. By some estimates, as many as 80 to 90 percent of patients seen in primary care practices have an associated affective mood disorder—anxiety, depression, or both.

The cost in lost productivity, damaged relationships with loved ones, physical disease, and actual loss of life is staggering. Depression is the primary cause of suicide, which is the ninth leading cause of death in the United States. Approximately 30,000 Americans die every year as a result of suicide.

This does not include deaths from "accidents" that may have been more deliberate than not. Suicide is the third most common cause of death among adolescents and the second most common among young adults. Age is no protection, however. One quarter of all suicides occur in the elderly.

What Is Depression?

Everyone feels sad or blue on occasion. But depression, as a clinical disorder, is more than just passing feelings of sadness or discouragement. It can go on for months or even years. A person who is depressed loses not only energy, but interest and joy in living. To suffer from depression is to feel that everything is awful and that nothing is ever going to get any better. At its least, depression pulls a thin gray film over one's existence. At its worst, it suffocates its victims in a black cloud of hopelessness.

Signs and Symptoms

There are no clinical tests for depression. Diagnosis is made on the basis of observation and symptoms such as the following:

Thoughts, Feelings, and Perceptions

- Diminished interest or pleasure in activities that one formerly enjoyed

- Loss of sexual desire

- Feelings of hopelessness, worthlessness, or inappropriate guilt

- Problems with concentration, memory, or decision-making

- Recurrent thoughts of death or suicide

Behavior

- Crying spells and irritability or, at the other extreme, apathy

- Significant change in appetite or weight (compulsive eating or lack of appetite)

- Neglecting one's appearance and responsibilities

- Withdrawal from friends, family, and activities

- Sleep disturbance (either insomnia or sleeping too much)

Physical Symptoms

- Trembling and shaking or decreased reflexes

- Chronic fatigue or lack of energy

- Unexplained physical complaints such as headaches, backaches, and digestive problems

Depression is often itself a symptom of an organic disorder, the most common one being hypothyroidism. However, it should be noted that this relationship goes both ways. People who are depressed can develop hypothyroidism. Depression is also a symptom of many other conditions, including:

- Pneumonia and other infections

- Cushing's disease (a steroid-secreting tumor)

- Addison's disease (a disorder in which the adrenal glands underfunction)

- Brain tumors

- Pernicious anemia

For this reason, a diagnosis of depression might include consideration of possible organic causes. In the overwhelming number of cases, however, depression does not have an organic cause, although organic processes may be associated with it.

What Causes It?

People often become depressed following an unhappy event, such as the breakup of a relationship, the death of a loved one, or the loss of a job. Although this type of depression hurts, it is an understandable reaction to a painful situation, and it usually tends to fade away with time. Often, however, the reasons for depression are not so easy to discern. Depression that has no apparent cause is much harder to understand and can lead to a sense of loss of control that only makes the depression worse.

A person who is depressed loses not only energy, but interest and joy in living.

Psychological theories about the causes of depression vary. Cognitive psychologists, for example, believe that depression arises from a negative view of the world caused by distorted perceptions and reasoning. In other words, depression results from the conflict between a person's view of how the world should be and how it actually is, or rather, how she perceives it to be. Another theory is that depression is "anger turned inward." Both of these theories, as well as many others, characterize depression as a response to irresolvable internal conflict. Another way of looking at it is to imagine two rams continually battering each other, each fighting for dominance. Because they are equally powerful, neither can dominate for long. Instead, they only succeed in negating and depleting each other's energy. If these two rams are opposing tendencies in an individual, such as a battle between "shoulds" and "wants," no wonder the person is exhausted and unhappy!

One way to view depression is as a withdrawal from intolerable stress, either physical, psychological, or both.

These internal conflicts can be compounded by added stressors, such as personality, environmental factors, illness, certain drugs (including alcohol), or diet. One way to view depression is as a withdrawal from intolerable stress, either physical, psychological, or both. You have probably heard of the "fight or flight" syndrome, which was first described in the 1930s. When confronted with perceived danger, an animal—human or otherwise—undergoes a physiological response that prepares her to defend herself or escape. She becomes more alert as epinephrine and steroid hormones pour through her system. Her heart and lungs work harder, pumping extra blood and oxygen to her muscles and brain, priming them for action. Immune cells pour into her bloodstream. All unnecessary functions—particularly the digestive system—are put on hold to permit the organism to deal with the immediate crisis. When the danger is passed, the alarm turns off, and all systems return to normal.

The relationship among mental, emotional, and physical health is not linear, based on simple cause-and-effect or a one- or two-way connection. It is more circular, with no boundaries to tell us where the physical leaves off and the emotional or mental begins.

This process was useful in the days when humans lived in a world where physical danger was an occasional, but intense reality. In our fast-paced, high-anxiety age, however, the process has become maladaptive. For most of us, physical danger is relatively rare, but psychological danger is pervasive.

Take, for instance, the worker who is dealing with an imminent deadline, impatient clients, or a demanding boss. To the body-mind, such a situation signals danger, and the person responds physiologically as if there were a lion in the room. Although the worker has the wisdom not to fight and believes that flight could bring greater danger (such as unemployment), she stays in a constant state of hyperalertness.

This inability to turn off the fight or flight response taxes every bodily system, from the brain and major organs, down to the cellular and even the molecular level. The effects at first are relatively insignificant, ranging from mood swings, to increased susceptibility to ailments like colds and flu, to minor accidents such as cutting a finger or banging a knee on the bed frame. As time goes on and the stress continues, its toll on the person increases. She may begin to suffer from such afflictions as:

- Tension and migraine headaches

- TMJ syndrome

- Gastroesophageal reflux

- Peptic ulcer disease

- Irritable bowel syndrome

- Constipation

- Hemorrhoids

- Depression

It is well known that chronic disease or severe trauma can lead to depression. However, recent evidence is showing that this is a two-way street. We are becoming more and more aware that depression can lead to chronic disease. The relationship among mental, emotional, and physical health is not linear, based on simple cause and effect or a one- or two-way connection. It is more circular, with no boundaries to tell us where the physical leaves off and the emotional or mental begins. Our minds are not simply passengers in our bodies. Each of us is a complex, wholly integrated mind-body system, and every part affects every other part in ways we are barely beginning to comprehend.

During the past thirty years, this realization has sparked a fascinating new field of research called psychoneuroimmunology (PNI). PNI has demonstrated at many different levels the intimate connection between a psychic process and a physiologic response, and vice versa. In particular, it has shown the dominant role that stress plays in every type of disease, whether a given condition is considered "physical" or "mental."

The Myth of a "Chemical Depression"

Over the past three decades experts have given increasing attention to the mechanism of depression. Although too complex to discuss in detail here, the research has focused on the workings of the brain, particularly the roles of neurotransmitters and brain hormones in various brain and body functions.

Neurotransmitters are molecules that transmit chemical information within the brain and from the brain to the other parts of the body. The association between neurotransmitter levels and mood has been well documented, although it is not yet understood. In depression, norepinephrine levels go down; in mania they go up. Low levels of serotonin are also associated with depressed mood. These observations have filtered through to the general public as the concept of "chemical depression." People think that for some unknown reason, neurotransmitter levels are thrown out of whack, thus resulting in depression. So what scientists regarded as a mechanism for viewing the workings of the brain has become transformed into a cause-and-effect relationship. This is sloppy thinking, however. Correlation is not the same as cause and effect. It can just as easily be theorized that depression causes changes in neurotransmitter levels as the other way around.

The idea that depression might have a purely physical cause, and a purely physical solution (in the form of antidepressants), has given patients who so desire (and there are many) the opportunity to relinquish control of their disease.

Nevertheless, research into the workings of the brain has led to a panoply of drugs that affect neurotransmitter levels and mood. This includes antidepressants, which are effective in elevating mood and reducing stress in both those suffering from depression and those who have to endure depression's infectious atmosphere. However, these medications may also be to depression what narcotics are to pain—habit-forming and a way to mask the underlying process.

I have heard far too many requests for antidepressants from patients who are unwilling to look at the underlying causes of their depression, because they are convinced that they have a unique illness called "chemical depression." The idea that depression might have a purely physical cause, and a purely physical solution (in the form of antidepressants), has given patients who so desire (and there are many) the opportunity to relinquish control of their disease. The recognition that there is a relationship between the chemical activity of the brain and a person's moods and behavior represents a critical step in our understanding of the workings of the human mind and body. But to interpret this correlation as cause and effect automatically negates the part of ourselves that is the mover and controller, that is, our spirit. The price of this negation is to relinquish freedom and personal power.

This is not to say that antidepressants don't serve a valuable purpose. They relieve the immediate pain and restore a person's ability to function. Hopefully, they also give people the energy and motivation to uncover and deal with the underlying causes of the depression. As we shall see, SAMe can also be of value in this process. But as we look at the various treatments for depression, remember that pills, whether they be conventional or alternative, are only dealing with the symptoms of depression, not its cause.

CHAPTER 8

CONVENTIONAL TREATMENTS FOR DEPRESSION

Most of the existing treatments for depression fall into two major realms: antidepressant drugs and psychotherapy. Within these broad categories are a wide array of options. Nearly all of them have merit in dealing with various aspects of this prevalent and often debilitating disease. However, the fact that there are so many treatments is a good indicator that none of them are specifically or enduringly effective.

I believe that the best therapy for depression—in fact, for any disease—is a multifaceted approach that works both to alleviate symptoms and to deal with the underlying causes. Thus, the best regimen is one that includes two components:

• Antidepressants to relieve the symptoms

• Psychotherapy to resolve the underlying conflicts that are causing the depression

I'll discuss how SAMe can fit into this picture in the next chapter.

Antidepressants

As society has become aware of the toll that depression takes on individuals, families, and the culture at large, the search has intensified for a treatment that is fast, cheap, and efficient. This in turn, has focused attention on mood-manipulating drugs, with profound—and in some ways alarming—implications.

Pharmacological treatments for anxiety and depression first came into vogue during the 1960s, when Valium and other tranquilizers were the drugs of choice. Since then, a multitude of more effective and less dangerous drugs has come into the marketplace. These new drugs were considered to be major breakthroughs because of their mood-altering effects and their relative safety. Antidepressants work fairly quickly, and their side effects are better tolerated with each new generation of drugs. Most notably, these new drugs relieve the immediate pain of depression and alter behavior enough to allow people to function in society. In fact, these drugs are so effective—and so easy to take—that many physicians consider them to be the main and only necessary treatment for mood disorders.

For most people, depression is mild and self-limiting, so dealing with it on a deeper level by addressing the causes is unnecessary from a medical care standpoint. To do so would be time-consuming, costly, and unreliable, as the success of psychotherapy depends in large part on both the skill of the therapist and the willingness of the patient to explore areas previously unseen and most likely painful to examine. Against the backdrop of modern medical care, where the primary goals are to limit costs and relieve symptoms, psychotherapy appears to be an expensive luxury. Granted, this battle is still being fought in managed care institutions and state legislatures, but the trend is definitely toward quick and efficient treatment for emotional problems rather than a longer, costlier attempt to transform a patient's thoughts, behavior, and approach to the world. Most patients actually support this view. The desire to relieve oneself of the numbing pain of depression prompts people to demand immediate relief.

That being said, let's look at the current chemical options for treating depression. Most of these fall into three general categories: tricyclics, selective serotonin re-uptake inhibitors (SSRIs), and MAO inhibitors.

Tricyclic Antidepressants

The tricyclics are so named due to their chemical structure, which has three rings connected side by side. As with so many drugs, we don't know exactly how tricyclics work. One theory is that they help raise levels of norepinephrine and serotonin in the brain by inhibiting their re-uptake into nerve endings, where they would be stored and thus out of circulation. Since low levels of these neurotransmitters are associated with depression, raising them can result in improved mood.

The most common tricyclics include:

- Imipramine
- Amitriptyline
- Desipramine
- Doxepin
- Nortriyptyiline

All of these have been around for quite some time. In fact, one advantage of the tricyclics over other types of antidepressants is that they have been around long enough to be available in generic form and are relatively inexpensive. They have been shown to be beneficial in those who tolerate them, which, unfortunately, leaves out a lot of people. It takes about three weeks for a patient to start realizing the antidepressant benefits of a tricyclic. Additionally, many clinicians start patients on the medication slowly in order to minimize potential adverse reactions. This could discourage an already stressed patient. Despite this cautious approach, various effects of these drugs prevent many people from ever reaching the appropriate dosage.

Tricyclics can be used selectively to treat specific depressive symptoms. For instance, a patient who complains of insomnia can be given amitriptyline or imipramine, both of which have sedating qualities. For someone who is a hypersomniac (sleeping all the time), desipramine is a better initial choice. Doxepin is right in the middle. Using the proper drug in a slowly progressive dose offers the greatest possibility that a patient will tolerate the drug and continue using it long enough for the antidepressant effects to become evident.

Side Effects of Tricyclics   Actually, the term "side effects" is something of a misnomer when referring to tricyclics or any other drug. By definition, a side effect is an effect other than the one the treatment is expected to have. An effect that is useful for treating one condition may be an unwanted side effect when treating a different condition. In each case, the effect is a natural result of using the drug. Whether it is beneficial, harmful, or neutral depends on the patient and his condition.

Unfortunately, many of the tricyclic effects are neither desired nor tolerated in a large percentage of patients. The *Physician's Desk Reference* lists so many adverse effects for tricyclics that it would not surprise me if most clinicians avoided their use altogether. If I had not seen for myself the benefits some people get from tricyclics, I would be reluctant to prescribe them.

I believe the best therapy for depression—in fact, for any disease— is a multifaceted approach that works both to alleviate symptoms and to deal with the underlying causes.

The most common side effects are blurry vision, dry mouth, constipation, weight loss or gain, and urinary retention. Another possible side effect is low blood pressure, resulting in light-headedness and fainting. This can be a problem for someone taking antihypertensive agents (for high blood pressure). Many people complain of a heavy "druggy" feeling. Less common are rashes or hives and itching. Men have been known to develop enlarged breasts, testicular swelling, and decreased libido or sexual desire. Women can also experience changes in their breasts and libido.

Dangerous but rare side effects associated with tricyclics include jaundice and hepatitis. Seizures can also occur, especially with overdose. The most serious potential consequence of tricyclic use is a propensity for abnormal heart conduction, a problem that results in irregular cardiac rhythms. Since these can be life threatening, anyone with heart problems should be especially cautious about using tricyclics. Doxepin has been shown to be safer for persons susceptible to heart arrhythmia. The effect of tricyclics during pregnancy and lactation is also a concern, and pregnant or nursing women should be carefully monitored while using them.

As with other drugs, the best way to determine whether a tricyclic is causing a particular effect is to discontinue the drug and see if the effect goes away. This should be done only under medical supervision, however, as stopping abruptly can cause withdrawal problems.

Selective Serotonin Re-Uptake Inhibitors

The most recent entrants—and current champions—in the antidepressant sweepstakes are the selective serotonin re-uptake inhibitors (SSRIs), which work similarly to the tricyclics. Both the medical and lay press have reported that SSRIs are the best thing for depression to date. Although SSRIs were originally believed to have significantly fewer side effects than the tricyclics, more recent studies have shown similar side effect profiles for both categories of drugs. Nevertheless, SSRIs are currently very popular with patients. This has come about partly due to their perceived effects, but also as a consequence of the limitations placed on reimbursement for psychotherapy. The need for purely symptomatic treatment of depression is well addressed with the new group of SSRI medications.

Fluoxetine, commonly known as Prozac, is the most popular SSRI. In many patients, Prozac has been effective in reducing depressive symptoms as well as in controlling the symptoms of obsessive-compulsive disorder and bulimia nervosa. As a rule, it does not cause drowsiness. In fact, people whose depressive symptoms include fatigue and hypersomnia particularly like Prozac. In rare cases, it reduces a man's ability to ejaculate, which can work in favor of one who has problems with premature ejaculation.

Like the tricyclics, SSRIs take about three weeks to become effective. The benefits are generally the same. In fact, there have been several studies comparing both the antidepressant effects and the side effects of SSRIs and tricyclics. The results are surprisingly similar for onset of action and frequency of side effects. This should prompt clinicians to try the older drugs before going on to the newer—and considerably more expensive—SSRIs.

Side Effects of SSRIs   The general side effects are essentially the same for all the SSRIs, with some individual peculiarities. The most frequent side effects are

• Nausea (23 percent of patients)

• Headaches (21 percent)

• Insomnia (20 percent)

   Less frequent symptoms, affecting around 10 percent of patients, are anxiety, nervousness, sleepiness, diarrhea, weakness, anorexia (loss of appetite), dry mouth, dizziness, tremors, stomach pains, and sweating. A small number of patients experience other symptoms including muscle pain, sore throat, decreased libido, rash, flatulence, vomiting, vision abnormalities, fever, and palpitations.

Prozac can be dangerous when combined with certain other drugs, particularly the anticoagulant Coumadin and MAO inhibitors. The amino acid tryptophan can enhance some of the symptoms associated with Prozac, especially agitation, restlessness, and gastrointestinal (GI) symptoms. Prozac does not show the obvious ill effects in pregnancy that the tricyclics do, and is probably the better choice during pregnancy. It can cause GI and sleep disturbances in infants, and it should not be used by nursing mothers.

Against the backdrop of modern medical care, where the primary goals are to limit costs and relieve symptoms, psychotherapy appears to be an expensive luxury.

Prozac has been blamed for some more dramatic and dangerous side effects, including suicidal tendencies. This allegation followed a report in the medical literature that observed that some people on Prozac had, in fact, committed suicide. Although the suicide rate for people on Prozac did not exceed that of the general population, this did not deter some individuals from pursuing, and sometimes winning, Prozac-related court cases.

The truth is that some people commit suicide soon after starting on antidepressants of any kind. This is hardly surprising. Depression can be so debilitating that any positive action seems impossible. The emotional boost that comes from starting antidepressants can provide just enough new energy that a person will, if disposed to do so, use it to end his life. I remember one particularly sad case of a woman who had been severely depressed for years. When she came to me, I discovered that her thyroid functions were far below normal. Within weeks of beginning appropriate doses of thyroid medication, she was discovered face down in a local lake. I can only surmise that she could no longer put up with a depression that had lasted perhaps for decades, even though it looked as though her nightmare would soon end.

In summary, Prozac and the other SSRIs are effective for relieving the symptoms of depression. Other drugs in this group include sertraline (Zoloft) and paroxetine (Paxil). These medications are interchangeable; a patient who does not tolerate one may try using another to increase antidepressant benefits or decrease side effects.

Monoamine Oxidase Inhibitors

Monoamine oxidase (MAO) is an enzyme that is produced in the brain and liver and that is used to metabolize the neurotransmitters norepinephrine, serotonin, and dopamine. Inhibiting the enzyme, therefore, helps maintain higher levels of these neurotransmitters, which can be a benefit in depression.

The MAO inhibitors were among the first antidepressants, dating back to the 1950s. Examples include isocarboxazid, phenelzine, and tranylcypromine.

Side Effects of MAOs   Unfortunately, high levels of norepinephrine can raise blood pressure, causing potentially fatal hypertension. This discovery considerably diminished the initial popularity of MAOs. Researchers later discovered that eating tyramine-rich foods greatly increases norepinephrine levels, and that reducing or eliminating these foods decreases the risk of hypertensive crises. Foods more likely to contain tyramine are those that are either aged or fermented, such as cheeses, beer, wine, yeast, pickled herring, and other pickled foods. Other foods that contain tyramine include chicken livers, broad beans, and coffee.

Some patients with severe or poorly responsive depression (so-called "atypical depressives") can do well on the MAO inhibitors. However, due to their significant shortcomings, most professionals refer patients who require MAOs to clinicians who have more experience prescribing them.

Other Antidepressants

In addition to the three major categories of antidepressants, there is a group of dissimilar medications that are loosely lumped under the term "heterocyclics":

- Wellbutrin (Bupropion)

- Effexor (Venlafaxine)

- Desyrel (Trazodone)

- Remeron (Mirtazapine)
- Serzone (Nefazodone)

Of these, bupropion is the most popular. It was on the market some years before Prozac and probably would be used just as widely were it not for the recognition that it can cause seizures. This side effect is unlikely, as long as it is used cautiously. Under the name Zyban, bupropion has been marketed as a smoking cessation aid, and studies demonstrate that it does reduce the craving for cigarettes. However, as with any addiction, the person still must be highly motivated to quit.

Electroconvulsive Therapy

Electroconvulsive therapy (ECT) is the most draconian treatment available for depression. It is generally reserved for patients who are so depressed that they are virtually incapacitated. It is also used for severely delusional patients, those with extreme agitation associated with depression, and patients with serious obsessive-compulsive disorders.

In ECT, two electrically conductive pads are placed on the anesthetized patient's temples and a strong current is run through his brain. This process appears to somehow push the brain's "reset" button and restore the person to normal functioning. Little is known about how or why ECT works. One theory is that the shock brings about mini-seizures that cause the therapeutic effect. ECT has brought people back from the brink of disaster to normal functioning.

The adverse effects include nausea, vomiting, fractures when relaxation is inadequate, and short-term memory loss.

The latter is the most controversial effect. Many patients who have undergone ECT claim that the resulting memory loss and inability to think clearly can last for years, even indefinitely. Given the risk of suicide associated with depression, and the fact that ECT can help allay this risk, it is sometimes necessary. Nevertheless, it should be used only in extreme cases, and then with great caution.

A skilled therapist will vary his approach and technique to the individual and the situation—sometimes supporting, sometimes drawing out information, sometimes challenging dysfunctional beliefs or habits.

Psychotherapy

Psychotherapy uses a process of talking and listening to help people bring about changes in their thinking, moods, and behavior. Virtually all psychotherapeutic approaches have in common fundamental principles relating to the workings of the unconscious mind. The unconscious is that part of our mind that we do not consciously perceive, but that nonetheless affects our behavior, mood, overt thinking, and even autonomic processes such as breathing, circulation, metabolism, and digestion. It is the repository of many of our prejudices, beliefs, and attitudes about life. An example of how the unconscious may work lies in this illustration: A three-year-old child is riding a tricycle on the sidewalk. A car rushes past, startling the child so she falls over. From then on, without any recollection of this incident, she becomes anxious whenever a car rushes past her. We all live with many such tapes in our unconscious mind. These tapes can cause us to respond inappropriately to present events or situations, because we unconsciously associate them with experiences we have long since forgotten.

Psychotherapy Techniques

Therapists have many different techniques for helping people resolve the inner conflicts that deplete energy and promote depression. A skilled therapist will vary his approach and technique to the individual and the situation—sometimes supporting, sometimes drawing out information, sometimes challenging dysfunctional beliefs or habits. With a skillful therapist and a committed client, such work can lead to positive outcomes, such as greater insight, less internal conflict, and increased self-confidence.

One of the most successful approaches for treating depression combines cognitive and behavioral techniques. Cognitive therapy focuses on how our thinking affects our behavior and emotions, and seeks to make people aware of errors or distortions in their thought processes. An example of such distorted thinking includes "all or nothing" thinking, where a person sees everything in absolutes: "If I do not do this perfectly, I will be a total failure." Another type of distorted thinking is a tendency to discount positive experiences, such as a compliment, while focusing on negative events. This type of thinking reinforces the person's negative perception of himself and the world around him.

> *[Philosopher–counselors] seek to put personal problems into a philosophical context, either by showing how a behavior or belief is inconsistent with a person's own observations, or by showing that the person's logic is internally inconsistent.*

If traumatic events are overshadowing a person's life, the cognitive approach examines how such events are interpreted by that person. The process becomes a sharing of perceptions between therapist and client. When they reach a common understanding of an event, the shared understanding makes it easier for the patient to acknowledge and process possibly faulty perceptions. The cognitive approach is more likely to succeed when both people hold similar systems of belief. It becomes more difficult, for instance, when a devout Christian is paired with a stolid atheist.

The behavioral approach encourages people to do new things, or do the same things differently, in order to change their perspective on life. These can be small changes, such as changing the style of one's hair, or major changes, such as changing one's job or career. The underlying principle is that a person develops his attitudes through his behavior, and that positive behavioral changes lead to similar changes in beliefs and attitudes.

Another approach seeks to give a depressed person insight into his emotions, particularly those he is repressing. People often repress or bury emotions in an unconscious attempt to protect themselves from pain. Such hidden, repressed emotions are the source of most psychosomatic diseases. The intense effort required to keep the emotional force hidden from one's own perception disrupts the body-mind, causing the conflict to appear in the form of physical symptoms. Therapy focused on exposing and resolving these volatile emotions leads patients to improved mood and elimination of their somatic symptoms.

An example of this is a patient I will call Nina, who suffered from tension headaches that became steadily worse throughout the day. I call this type of headache the Atlas Syndrome, after the Greek god who bore the world on his shoulders. Nina felt it was her duty to carry the responsibilities of everyone in her household. Although outwardly calm, she resented her burden. Therapy helped Nina recognize the depth of her resentment and gave her the courage to change her behavior. When she began doing only what she saw as appropriate and delegated responsibilities to other members of her family, her headaches ceased. Nina's challenge was to over-come her fear that if she stopped taking care of them, her family would stop loving her.

Alternatives to Psychotherapy

Conventional medicine sees depression as a disease to be cured, controlled, or hidden. Even psychotherapy often deals with thoughts and emotions in isolation rather than in the context of a person's life. Modern therapeutic approaches work so hard at not imposing the therapist's values on the patient, that sometimes the process leaves a person feeling more upbeat, but not substantially changed. I am reminded of a joke about a man who entered a bar and ordered a beer. When the bartender placed it in front of him, he downed it, then proceeded to punch the bartender in the nose. He was immediately remorseful, exclaiming, "I don't understand this compulsion. Every time I drink a beer, I must punch someone. I feel terrible!"

The bartender was mollified by this explanation, and advised him to see a psychiatrist to deal with this problem. The drinker accepted the advice and promptly left. The following month, the man went into the same bar and ordered a beer. The bartender was quick to comply. Having finished the draft, the man promptly punched the bartender again.

"Didn't you see the psychiatrist, like I asked you to?" asked the bartender, rubbing his sore proboscis.

"Yes. I did," said the man, "I still have the compulsion. I just don't feel guilty about it anymore."

Of course not all psychotherapy lacks such context. Many discursive therapies work within a specific context, and there are plenty of therapists whose approach takes into account the basic beliefs of their clients. These include both traditional religious counseling, and the new, but growing practice of philosophical counseling.

Religious Counseling

Religious counseling, whatever the creed involved, has at its base a view of the world as having a spiritual and moral center. This provides a structural context within which the patient can work to resolve his or her depression. For example, if duty to God is the foundation of one's beliefs, then it is inappropriate to live primarily for one's own happiness. In such a case, depression is a result of the conflict arising from not acting according to the tenets of one's faith. In the hypothetical situation above, if the person puts her own happiness before duty to God, depression stems from the schism between how she lives and how she believes she should live. The depressed person can lessen, or even resolve, her internal conflict by bringing her behavior in line with the rules laid down in her belief structure. The objective is not to find happiness, but to achieve greater harmony between how she lives and what she believes. Ironically, doing so can resolve the depression and lead to greater happiness. This approach underscores the multifaceted nature of the human spirit, which requires many elements to work together for a functioning, balanced whole.

Philosophical Counseling

Many people, however, do not accept the existence of a divine unifying force or do not subscribe to a specific set of religious beliefs. For such people, a religious contextual approach would be decidedly unhelpful, even repugnant. However, during the last few years, a new type of therapist has appeared—the philosophical counselor. These counselors are trained philosophers who contend that depression and other mood disorders are the result of philosophical confusion. Philosopher–counselors contend that psychiatry and psychology have failed the people that they serve: first, by merely alleviating symptoms; and second, by ignoring the moral and social context of individual problems. These therapists seek to put personal problems into a philosophical context, either by showing how a behavior or belief is inconsistent with a person's own observations, or by showing that the person's logic is internally inconsistent. The idea is that recognition of such inconsistencies will bring about changes in the person's thinking and approach to the world, and will consequently result in changes in his behavior. This will resolve the internal conflict and alleviate the depression.

As an example of how philosophical counseling might work, imagine a fictitious person named Michael who became a lawyer for idealistic reasons. He intended to right wrongs, defend the innocent, and remedy injustices. Years of practicing law have brought him to the point where he is suffering from a siege mentality brought on by trying to maintain his ideals in the face of a world that, as evidenced by its actions, does not want what he has to offer—at least not in the way he had anticipated. As a result of the ongoing conflict between what he thinks reality should be and what he believes it is, he gets depressed.

Michael could go to a psychologist, who might talk about the different frustrations that he's having and offer some support and insights into what he is feeling. He could take an antidepressant, which may or may not help his mood, and most likely would only mask his symptoms while the nagging doubts about his work persist. Instead, he goes to a philosophical counselor. The philosopher examines Michael's situation and discovers his idealism. The philosopher points out that the world in which Michael lives is rather different from what he imagines it is. That is, he believes that the purpose of the legal system is to dispense justice, but in reality it is a utilitarian system that exists primarily to settle disputes.

. . . the right combination of medicine and psychotherapy can help people overcome even the most desperate levels of depression.

The philosopher's task is to help Michael realize that the problem is not that the world is against him, but rather that the world has a different view of things than he does. Seeing this conflict in a philosophical way enables Michael to choose how he wants to approach his problem. Since philosophy works in a logical realm, he gets to make logical choices:

1. He can accept that this is the way the world is and that it neither will change nor wants to change. He can then change his own philosophy and adopt the utilitarian approach of settling disputes.

2. He can use his insights to establish some inroads with the people with whom he deals, by showing the utilitarian value of achieving justice, both immediately and in the long term.

3. He can opt out altogether by leaving the profession and doing something different in which his ideals will not be so compromised.

Any of these choices is viable, as long as he has the logical capabilities to perceive his problem, the courage to follow through with his decision, and the patience to accept the changes he will need to make in order to satisfy the conditions of his choice.

Which Approach Is Best?

There are many variations on these approaches, too many to cover here. Virtually all psychotherapies have something to offer the explorer of the human psyche, and both chemical and psychotherapeutic treatments have the potential to help patients suffering from depression. Should one choose to delve into the psychological factors underlying his depression, it is not so much an issue of choosing the right approach as one of choosing an appropriate therapist and having the will and courage to see the process through.

Unfortunately, in most medical circles, discussions about depression and anxiety are limited to their bodily manifestations. The focus is on somatic effects, neurological mechanisms, and of course, pharmacological treatment. Psychiatrists do less and less counseling and more drug treatment. Many clinicians believe that depression is a self-limiting disorder that will eventually go away by itself, much like a bad cold or a muscle strain. Even more common is the supposition that depression is essentially a chemical phenomenon that can be corrected by chemical intervention. Although at some level, medications can reduce the pain of depression, they do nothing to alter the cause. However, the right combination of medicine and psychotherapy can help people overcome even the most desperate levels of depression. As we've seen, conventional medications carry with them risks and undesirable effects, which leaves the door open for alternative treatments, including SAMe.

CHAPTER 9

SAMe AND OTHER ALTERNATIVE TREATMENTS FOR DEPRESSION

A s we saw in the last chapter, antidepressant medications can do much to alleviate the symptoms of depression. As with many drugs, however, the balance between benefits and risks is a precarious one. After all, a primary goal in treating depression is to improve the sufferer's quality of life. A 1950s commercial asked, "Why trade a headache for an upset stomach?" The same can be said of antidepressants. Why trade depression for nausea, headache, insomnia, anxiety, nervousness, somnolence, diarrhea, weakness, anorexia, dry mouth, dizziness, tremor, stomach pain, sweating, muscle pain, sore throat, decreased libido, rash, flatulence, vomiting, yawning, itching, abnormal vision, fever, or palpitations? Shouldn't there be some other options?

There are, in fact, a number of them. The effects of alternative treatments, including SAMe, may not be as dramatic as some of the treatments we've already discussed, especially electroconvulsive therapy. However, as we will see, alternative treatments have many benefits that the conventional treatments cannot match. As a group, they are gentler. Some can be more enduring. Like SAMe, they may reduce the symptoms of depression with fewer side effects. Or, like religious or philosophical counseling, they may provide a context that enables a person to find a road out of depression, toward a better way of life.

Using SAMe for Depression

SAMe's neurophysiological effects are not as readily apparent as its effects on joint physiology. What we do know is incomplete. In all fairness, however, we have little real knowledge about how any antidepressants work. We do know that norepinephrine and serotonin play a role in depression, and that SAMe, as a methyl donor, plays a significant part in the production of these neurotransmitters. SAMe levels have also been shown to be markedly decreased in patients with severe depression.[1] Patients who receive either oral or intravenous doses of SAMe show marked rises in the level of SAMe in their cerebrospinal fluid. This indicates that exogenous SAMe is capable of crossing the blood-brain barrier and being used by the brain.

SAMe and the Brain

So how might SAMe relate to depression? One possibility has to do with the production of phospholipids, a necessary constituent of cell membranes. One theorist suggests that depression occurs when the membranes of nerve cells are unable to accept the proper neurotransmitters, and that SAMe may function by affecting the consistency of the membranes and making them more responsive to stimulation.[2] An expansion of this theory infers that many neurological and psychiatric dysfunctions relate to impaired methylation at several areas, including the cell membranes, the receptor sites, and neurotransmitter production.[3]

After all, a primary goal in treating depression is to improve the sufferer's quality of life.

SAMe appears to have an intriguing relationship with melatonin, another supplement that has been in the news lately. Melatonin is a hormone that is found in two places in the brain: the pituitary and the pineal glands. Research over the past two decades has shown that melatonin production is inhibited in the presence of light and enhanced in darkness. This has led to some insights regarding seasonal depression (seasonal affective disorder or SAD) and time-related mood disorders such as jet lag. Research indicates that SAMe and melatonin levels in the pineal glands have an inverse relationship—when melatonin levels are down, SAMe levels are up, and vice versa.[4] This has raised some interest in the relationship of both SAMe and melatonin levels to depression (there is no evidence to support the use of melatonin for treating depression).

Not surprisingly, it also adds another twist to the complexity of the biochemical aspects of depression.

Some studies have shown that SAMe levels are depleted by the use of tricyclic antidepressants, and SAMe has been shown to be effective on people with recurrent depression who were not responsive to tricyclics.[5-7] SAMe also appears to stimulate production of dopamine, a neurotransmitter that plays a major role in Parkinson's disease.[8] I'll discuss this more in Chapter 12.

All these studies seem to imply that SAMe has more than one route of activity in the brain and that it works on improving mood in ways that are different from the antidepressants that are presently on the market. This may explain why SAMe can work alongside an antidepressant to hasten the onset of mood improvement.

Clinical Effects of SAMe on Depression

The effects of SAMe on depression were seen as early as 1972.[9] In 1978, researchers studying the potential effect of SAMe on schizophrenia noticed that many patients' moods improved even though their schizophrenic symptoms, such as hallucinations, did not.[10] Over the years, other studies have trickled in regarding SAMe's potential antidepressant effects. Although they sparked some mild interest, the studies remained sparse, using small patient groups. They were large enough in most instances, however, to demonstrate statistical significance. I should note that most studies regarding the effects of antidepressants are small and of short duration. This is true of studies involving the tricyclics and SSRIs as well as SAMe.

It wasn't until publication of a meta-analysis of all the pre-1994 studies that a clearer picture of SAMe's antidepressant capabilities emerged.[11] You'll recall from Chapter 3 that a meta-analysis is a process whereby a number of related studies are combined and analyzed as a group. The larger grouping helps to clarify the findings in the smaller studies. This is especially important if the studies are numerous and small, as in the case of SAMe and depression, or when the individual studies contradict each other.

Patient responses to treatment were measured using the Hamilton Depression Scale (HAM-D), an interview tool used by psychologists and psychiatrists to rate the extent and severity of depression. The baseline on the HAM-D scale identifies all the elements, or symptoms, of depression. Resolution of 25 to 49 percent of these symptoms is considered a partial response. Resolution of 50 percent or more of the symptoms is considered a full response.

Meta-analysis—Uncontrolled Trials

There were 377 subjects in 13 uncontrolled trials. These were studies that reviewed patients' response to SAMe over a period of time, without comparing their responses to patients on placebos or other drugs. The duration of the studies ranged from eight to 42 days. The dosage of SAMe was from 45 to 135 mg intramuscularly (IM), 60 to 350 mg intravenously (IV), or 1,600 mg orally. The studies showed an overall positive response; even two of seven patients who had not responded to antidepressants showed a response to SAMe.[12] However, the lack of comparison groups makes these studies of limited scientific value.

Meta-analysis—Controlled Studies

The controlled studies involved a total of 793 participants.[13] Subjects and studies were removed from the meta-analysis if they did not fit its criteria. For example, a study was removed if it used measurement instruments that could not easily be compared with the other studies; for instance, if the researchers used a different tool than the HAM-D to measure patient responses. This left 198 patients for studies comparing SAMe with a placebo, and 201 patients for studies comparing SAMe with tricyclic antidepressants.

SAMe versus Placebos The SAMe versus placebo studies ranged in duration from 7 to 42 days. The dosages were 45 to 200 mg IM, 45 to 400 mg IV, and 1,600 mg orally per day. Of the six studies reported, five showed SAMe to have a greater response rate than the placebo. The largest two of these studies were statistically significant. The sixth study found little difference between SAMe and the placebo.

Overall, the partial response rate for SAMe was 70 percent, compared to 30 percent for the placebo. The full response rate was 38 percent for SAMe and 22 percent for the placebo. Broken down, these studies provide a much weaker case for SAMe versus placebo, with only two studies showing a significantly better response rate for SAMe, and three showing an equal or poorer response rate.

SAMe Versus Tricyclics The studies comparing SAMe and tricyclics lasted from 14 to 42 days. The tricyclics used were amitriptyline, chlorimipramine, imipramine, and desipramine, all in therapeutic doses. The dosages for SAMe were 200 to 400 mg IV or 1,600 mg orally per day. The partial response rates for both were very similar, at 92 percent for SAMe and 85 percent for the antidepressants. The full response rates were also similar, at 61 percent for SAMe and 59 percent for the tricyclics. More significant is the fact that these outcomes were fairly uniform for all of the studies.

Other Studies

Two other studies are worth noting, because of their findings regarding SAMe's rapid response time. In one study,[14] 195 patients given 400 mg IM of SAMe daily showed response in 7 to 14 days. This compares to a minimum of 21 days for other antidepressants (even longer for St. John's wort). The second study compared the onset of response to a combination of SAMe (200 mg IM/day) and the tricyclic imipramine (150 mg orally/day) versus imipramine alone. Depressive symptoms decreased more rapidly with the combination than with imipramine alone.[15]

Overall, the results of the research on SAMe and depression are both encouraging and limited. The biggest problem is the small number of studies. What is clear is that the existing evidence is encouraging enough to warrant further research. At the very least, it's worth considering using SAMe to "jumpstart" conventional antidepressants by combining both during the first two to three weeks of therapy. This is how SAMe is most commonly used in Europe.

How Much SAMe
Should You Take for Depression?

As with arthritis, taking SAMe orally seems to be as effective for depression as administering it intramuscularly or intravenously, and it avoids the whole problem of needles. Based on the available studies, I would recommend the following:

- Start with a dosage of 1,600 mg a day—either 800 mg twice a day or 400 mg four times a day—for about two or three weeks, or until you start to feel the antidepressant effects.

- Gradually reduce the dosage to 800 mg or even 400 mg a day, based on your depressive symptoms.

- Since evidence indicates that SAMe will not work when B12 and folate levels are low, it's a good idea to take these supplements while taking SAMe; one mg a day is sufficient.

When combining SAMe with an antidepressant, start off with the higher dose of SAMe (1,600 mg a day) and taper it down to a maintenance dose, or even stop it altogether once the antidepressant has had time to take effect. As I said before, SAMe probably uses multiple pathways in the brain, and at least one of these is a different route than those used by antidepressants. This means it might be possible to adjust the doses of SAMe and antidepressant simultaneously, using your symptoms as a guide.

Using SAMe at the same time as either an SSRI or a tricyclic (I prefer the tricyclics, because they're cheaper) might enable you to take a lower dose of the tricyclic, thus reducing unwanted side effects. Unfortunately there is just not enough information for us to really know how SAMe would work over a long period of time, either alone or combined with an antidepressant.

Herbs and Supplements

A number of herbs and supplements are reported to be effective for depression. For some of these, the evidence is merely anecdotal, while others have shown positive results in scientific studies.

St. John's wort

Probably the most well known and successful herb for treating depression is St. John's wort *(Hypericum)*. In study after study, St. John's wort has been shown to be an effective antidepressant as compared to placebos. It also compares favorably to imipramine, one of the tricyclic antidepressants. Using the HAM-D Scale, patients on St. John's wort showed a greater than 50 percent improvement in depressive symptoms. These studies included a total of 1,757 people in 23 clinical trials—no less significant than studies conducted for Prozac and the other SSRIs.

SAMe's neurophysiological effects are not as readily apparent as its effects on joint physiology. . . . In all fairness, however, we have little real knowledge about how any antidepressants work.

St. John's wort takes somewhat longer than the tricyclics and SSRIs to become effective—about four to six weeks. Compared to the chemical antidepressants, St. John's wort produces far fewer side effects and is reasonable in cost. However, because it is an herb, it does not fall under the regulation of the FDA. This means that you have no guarantee (and in fact, it is unlikely) that the St. John's wort capsules you buy at the health food store or your local supermarket contain the same formula, concentration, and purity as the St. John's wort used in the studies.

Valerian Root

Valerian root *(Valeriana officinalis)* has a mild sedating effect and is often used as a sleep aid. Though not directly an antidepressant, it has been a favorite of mine for treating anxiety symptoms for many years (over time, anxiety wears a person out and leads to depression). Indeed, valerian is as effective and considerably less habit-forming than Valium, the 1960s standby for anxiety and mild depression.

L-tryptophan and 5-HTP

As mentioned in Chapter 2, L-tryptophan is an essential amino acid found in many foods. Studies have shown that it is effective in alleviating anxiety and mild depression; it is also used as a sleep aid. L-tryptophan was popular in the 1980s, until the FDA banned its sale in 1988 because of an association with eosinophilic myalgia syndrome (EMS), a sometimes fatal illness. Subsequent study revealed that the cause of the syndrome was not tryptophan itself, but a contaminant that was limited to a process performed by a single laboratory in Japan. Despite this evidence, there have not been any attempts to make tryptophan widely available again in this country. I suspect this is because it would compete with the considerably more lucrative prescription anti-anxiety agents on the market.

L-tryptophan is currently available by prescription from a few compounding pharmacies in the United States. It is possible that it will eventually be available in the general American market, as it is increasingly being manufactured by pharmaceutical companies that adhere to more exacting standards. This new type of manufacturing could ease FDA anxieties about its safety, if that is truly the reason it was banned.

At the very least, it's worth considering using SAMe to "jumpstart" conventional antidepressants by combining both during the first two weeks of therapy.

Recently, a modified form of L-tryptophan called 5-hydroxytryptophan (5-HTP) became available in the United States. Unlike L-tryptophan, which is produced by a biological fermentation process, 5-HTP is derived from the seeds of a West African medicinal plant called *Griffonia simplicifolia.* 5-HTP is actually the next phase in the multi-step equation between L-tryptophan and serotonin. Once absorbed into the body, it is converted to serotonin. (As I mentioned in Chapter 7, low levels of serotonin are associated with depression and other mood disorders.) Preliminary evidence indicates that

5-HTP is effective in treating depression, comparing favorably with the tricyclics and SSRIs. Like L-tryptophan, it can also aid sleep. Some research indicates that 5-HTP may help promote weight loss by reducing carbohydrate cravings.

Non-Western Approaches

Practitioners of disciplines that fall outside the western medical model have been treating depression and its symptoms for many centuries. Chinese medicine, of which acupuncture is a part, has been very successful in this realm. In recent years, attempts have been made to study the effectiveness of such practices using a western scientific model. In one such study, acupuncture successfully reduced pain and enhanced sleep in over 90 percent of the subjects studied.[16]

Although an in-depth exploration of non-western treatments for depression is outside the scope of this book, a brief look at one such approach may provide an idea of how differently other cultures regard this common human condition. Ayurvedic medicine, the medical discipline practiced in India and Sri Lanka, takes a multifaceted approach to healing illnesses including depression. It recognizes that disease is manifested at all levels of the mind and body. According to Ayurveda, humans have three psychological qualities:

- *Satva,* the state of pure qualities, the essential nature of the person
- *Rajas,* the pleasure-seeking qualities of the soul
- *Tomas,* the animalistic, reactive, destructive qualities

Disorders occur when Rajas and Tomas overbalance Satva.

Treatment is negotiated between the healer and the patient. The healer, while recognizing the need for the patient to change his behavior, brings out the processes that are not in the patient's control. This includes such factors as social elements and cultural patterning; humoral changes (that is, metabolic, genetic, or other changes that are "built in" to the body); and communication habits. By putting together a holistic model of the patient's problem, the healer mitigates issues of personal responsibility, thus reducing the individual's natural tendency to defend himself instead of seeing all the causes of his illness.

Probably the most well known and successful herb for treating depression is St. John's wort (Hypericum).

The treatment has several processes:

- Certain medicines are used to help the symptoms, along with other natural elements such as minerals.

- Meditations are employed, including forms of suggestion and hypnosis, persuasion, and ritualistic therapy. In ritualistic therapy, symptoms are actually transferred—the patient can put her ills into another animal and release them. This is similar to the biblical and Talmudic new year practice in which a high priest transferred the sins of the nation onto a goat (azazel in Hebrew), then pushed the animal off a cliff to its death (thus the term "scapegoat").

- Atonement and rectification are also necessary elements of healing the disease.

- Finally, healthful practices are prescribed in the form of tantric and yogic exercises.

Interestingly, in Ayurvedic medicine, the healer's adherence to his own recommendations is considered more important than his knowledge of the art of healing. It makes sense to me that a person who heals will be more effective both as a healer and as a witness to the proper healing process if she practices what she preaches.

CHAPTER 10

SAMe AND
THE LIVER

Perhaps nowhere are SAMe's benefits so dramatic as in the liver. The evidence is sparse but compelling that SAMe can actually repair or reverse damage caused by cirrhosis of the liver—a progressive, degenerative disease for which transplantation is the only known effective treatment.

Meet the Liver

The liver is the body's largest organ, weighing about three pounds in the average adult. It is also one of the most interesting and complex organs, serving as the body's main chemical factory. Among its many important products are various blood proteins, urea, and cholesterol. The latter, despite its bad image in the media, is essential to life. It provides the basic structure for bile salts, which in turn are used to make bile, which is necessary for metabolizing fats. Cholesterol is also used to make steroids. These hormones, which are made by the adrenals and the gonads, are critical to many body processes. In addition to its manufacturing work, the liver stores fats and carbohydrates, helps regulate blood glucose levels, and stores iron and some vitamins. It also modifies steroidal hormones and inactivates many hormones in the body.

A key part of the liver's job is detoxification—breaking down poisonous substances into ones that can be easily used or passed out of the body.

A key part of the liver's job is detoxification—breaking down poisonous substances into ones that can easily be used or passed out of the body. These toxins include drugs, alcohol, and the body's own metabolic by-products and wastes. Because of this role, the liver is constantly in harm's way. It is a wonder that it survives at all, given the threats posed by environmental toxins and the various substances we voluntarily put into our bodies. Yet not only does it survive, it thrives. It is almost impossible to destroy the liver. Remove 80 percent of it, and it will regenerate to its original size in months. Transplant part of a liver, and barring complications, both the donor and the donated portions will grow to full size and functionality. As long as it retains its structural integrity, it can regrow like the tail of a tadpole. It is the only organ that can do this. By contrast, if you take away a piece of the heart or brain, it is gone forever.

But the liver is not invincible. If its structure is violated, it doesn't have a blueprint for regeneration. The liver, unlike the heart or the lungs or the brain, is actually a gland. It consists of cells that do the body's metabolic, or chemical work, along with channels that bring work to the cells and take the finished products away. When toxins damage this basic structure, blockages occur, preventing the free movement of enzymes and transformed toxins, which can then cause increased damage.

As we shall see, SAMe plays a critical role in protecting the integrity of the liver. This is true for both SAMe that is manufactured within the body and SAMe that enters the body from outside.

What Is Cirrhosis of the Liver?

Cirrhosis is a condition in which the liver gradually loses its ability to perform its primary functions. In essence, it is a slow death by poisoning, as the liver becomes unable to eliminate the toxins that come into or are manufactured by the body.

What Causes It?

At least 40 different conditions can cause cirrhosis of the liver. Most of them are relatively rare, at least in the United States. Some of the more common causes include the following:

- Damage from Hepatitis B and C

- Heart failure

- Biliary obstruction, in which the bile ducts are blocked by gallstones, scar tissue, or other obstructions

- Chronic pancreatitis, a condition commonly seen in alcoholics

- Overconsumption of alcohol

- Exposure to certain toxic chemicals

- A number of different drugs

Inherited conditions that can lead to cirrhosis include hemachromatosis, a metabolic disorder in which excess iron accumulates in the liver, pancreas, and other organs; and Wilson's disease, another metabolic disorder that causes the liver, brain, kidneys, and corneas to absorb too much copper. Cirrhosis of the liver can also be caused by an overdose of vitamin A, a potent reminder that not all supplements are necessarily safe, and that too much of a good thing can be bad for you. In fact, if taken in excessive amounts, all of the fat-soluble vitamins, including A, D, and E, can cause various problems with the liver and other organs.

In the United States, the leading cause of cirrhosis is chronic overconsumption of alcohol, which accounts for three-quarters of all cases. Alcoholic cirrhosis is found in 1.6 to 9.9 percent of all necropsy examinations performed in the United States, depending on which studies you use. Twice as many men are affected as women, and although it is most commonly seen in people 40 to 55 years old, it is not that unusual to find it in people in their twenties. As a medical student, I once saw the body of a 28- or 29-year-old man who already had an advanced case of cirrhosis with ascites. Ascites is a collection of fluid in the abdomen, which happens because a person's liver is so clogged up from the cirrhosis that fluid backs up into the abdomen. Despite his youth, this man had managed to literally drink himself to death.

How Much Is Too Much?

How much drinking does it take to cause cirrhosis of the liver? The actual amounts vary from one individual to another, but if you consume 40 to 80 grams of alcohol a day over a ten to fifteen year period, your chances of getting it are pretty well assured. This means 36 to 72 ounces of beer (three to six 12-ounce glasses), 4½ to 9 ounces of liquor (four to eight shots), or 15 to 30 ounces of wine (four to eight glasses).

Note that beer and wine "count" just as much as whisky or vodka. I have heard many people claim that they didn't drink too much because all they ever drank was beer. And as for wine, I remember one patient I'll call Edith. She was a quiet, gentle older woman, the very image of a "sweet little old lady." She had severe cirrhosis of the liver, but insisted all she ever had was a little bit of wine with dinner. It turned out that a "little bit of wine" was a full bottle, which she had consumed all by herself, every single night for years.

What Alcohol Does to the Liver

Since the liver is, in essence, a chemical factory, any damage to the liver is chemical damage, which takes place at a cellular level. You may remember from high school or college biology that all cells contain mitochondria. The mitochondria are the body's energy factories. They take in glucose and convert it into pure energy, which then gets transferred back into molecules that help to power the body. Alcohol reduces the ability of the mitochondria to accept substances, probably by poisoning the mitochondrion membrane.

That's not all. As the body's detoxifier, the liver converts ethanol (the alcohol in alcoholic beverages) into vinegar, a nontoxic substance that is easily used or passed out of the body. However, along the way, the liver first converts the ethanol to acetaldehyde, which is itself a toxic substance. It is during this intermediate step that the damage takes place. The acetaldehyde does three things:

- It decreases the ability of the kidneys to drain uric acid. This causes uric acid to accumulate in the body, which can contribute to gout—a good reason not to drink when you have gout.

- It decreases the liver's ability to convert fats into energy.

- It decreases the liver's ability to convert glycogen into glucose.

Remember that one of the liver's functions is to store fats and carbohydrates, in the form of fatty acids and glycogen, and convert them to energy and glucose as needed. When this conversion process is impaired, the liver cells become increasingly packed with fatty acids and glycogen. This puts pressure on the cells, eventually causing cell damage and disruption. The result is that the cells become unable to perform their functions, which includes detoxifying not only alcohol, but many other substances that come into the body, including drugs and by-products of metabolic processes. What happens then is a downward spiral of decreased cell function, which leads to cell damage, which leads to the liver's inability to do its job, especially to detoxify harmful substances and metabolize them into safe ones. As the liver cells clog up with fat, they become sluggish and bloated. This is called a "fatty liver"—the first step leading to cirrhosis.

Cirrhosis is a condition in which the liver gradually loses its ability to perform its primary functions. In essence, it is a slow death by poisoning . . .

If a person stops drinking at this point, there's a good chance that those cells that haven't completely lost their integrity can come back to a relatively normal state. Unfortunately, this is not what usually happens. The person keeps drinking, and the fatty liver causes the cells to break down even further. This process can be precipitated by other conditions such as those mentioned above. Whatever the cause, however, drinking alcohol will definitely make the condition worse.

From Fatty Liver to Cirrhosis

When the liver cells break down, like any damaged tissue, they begin to scar. The scarring becomes widespread and starts to contract, as scars do, which constricts the channels in the liver—that is, blood vessels and bile ducts. Because the blood vessels are impaired, the blood flow through the liver, which is significant, is impaired as well. This causes blood to back up into the spleen, the intestine, and even the legs, causing hemorrhoids and esophageal varices, which are like hemorrhoids or varicose veins in the esophagus. The pressure on the blood vessels eventually causes them to seep fluid, which leaks into the abdomen and possibly the legs as well. Because the blood vessels have thin walls and are under high pressure, they may break, causing internal bleeding in the upper stomach and esophagus, a potentially fatal event.

Alcoholic cirrhosis can ultimately lead to alcoholic hepatitis, in which the liver completely loses its ability to detoxify and becomes toxic itself.

Meanwhile, the liver is also losing its ability to produce proteins and bile. Because of the impaired bile ducts, the bile that is produced cannot be channeled out appropriately, so it actually causes even more harm to the liver. Because the liver can't make enough of the proteins needed for blood clotting, the person may bleed or bruise easily. Because the liver can't perform its detoxification functions properly, toxins build up in the blood, resulting in even more damage to the liver and other parts of the body, including the brain. Many of the signs that we associate with advanced alcoholism, such as neglect of one's appearance, forgetfulness, and confusion, may be due to the accumulation of toxins in the brain. Because drugs cannot be metabolized properly, the person with cirrhosis may also be extra-sensitive to medications and their effects.

In alcoholic cirrhosis, all of these problems are often compounded by poor nutrition, since many alcoholics get most of their nutrition from the alcohol itself. Thus, they are often deficient in vitamins, particularly B12 and folic acid.

Signs and Symptoms

Early symptoms of cirrhosis of the liver include fatigue, enlarged liver, nausea, and poor appetite. Often, however, the condition does not produce any symptoms until the liver is well along its way to total ruin. Alcoholic cirrhosis can ultimately lead to alcoholic hepatitis, in which the liver completely loses its ability to detoxify and becomes toxic itself. Symptoms of alcoholic hepatitis include:

- Weight loss

- Abdominal pain

- Vomiting

- Nausea

- Loss of appetite

- Enlarged and/or tender liver

- Jaundice (yellow eyes and skin)

- Fever

- Fluid accumulation in the abdomen (ascites) and legs

- Enlarged spleen

- Spider blood vessels

- Hair loss

- Breast enlargement in men

- Hallucinations

- Coma

People at this stage are also extremely susceptible to infection.

At the end stages of cirrhosis, the liver becomes unable to metabolize protein effectively. When this happens, eating too much protein can be fatal. This is because when the body can't metabolize protein, it breaks down into ammonia. Ammonia is a powerful poison. If the liver can't get rid of it, the person begins to hallucinate and eventually falls into a coma and dies. Thus, death from cirrhosis is often death by ammonia poisoning.

I remember one patient, a man named Jerry, who demonstrated this whole pattern of events. I first saw Jerry when he was hospitalized for pneumonia, by which time he already had well-advanced alcoholic cirrhosis and hepatitis. When I asked him how much he drank, he told me he had drunk a fifth of Southern Comfort every single day for the past 17 years.

I asked. "Why Southern Comfort?"

He said, "Because it's sweet, and I hate the taste of alcohol."

Jerry was in bad shape. I saw him three times in that rotation alone. It was November, and Thanksgiving was coming up. The week before Thanksgiving, he had improved enough to go home, so I sent him off with a warning not to eat any turkey for Thanksgiving. His liver was so far gone that I knew he would not be able to handle more than a tiny amount of protein.

The day after Thanksgiving, Jerry was back in the hospital, this time in a coma. I asked his wife what had happened. She said, "Well, he just ate a turkey leg."

"A turkey leg!" I exclaimed. "That's a lot of meat!"

She said, "It was a small turkey."

Humorous though this anecdote might be, the man died during this hospitalization.

Treatment

Conventional treatment for cirrhosis of the liver is limited and not very specific. It consists mainly of trying to manage the symptoms and compensate for nutritional deficiencies. This includes eating a well-balanced diet and taking supplements that include folate, thiamine, peridoxine, and vitamin K, as well as replacing magnesium and phosphate. Diuretics may be used to reduce fluid retention, and antibiotics may help to reduce ammonia build-up. In the case of an alcoholic, the person must stop drinking, so treatment may include psychological counseling or other treatment programs.

In some cases, cirrhosis of the liver may be cured by replacing the damaged liver with a new one—in other words—a transplant. For an alcoholic who insists on continuing to drink, however, this would be a waste of time, trouble, and society's as well as the individual's money.

SAMe and the Cirrhotic Liver

SAMe is abundant in the liver of a healthy person. In fact, that is where the greatest concentrations of SAMe are found. Among other things, SAMe has the ability to transfer sulfur, which is used to make cysteine, taurine, and glutathione, all important substances for metabolism. Taurine and glutathione, in particular, are required to make bile salts.

Since cirrhosis appears to limit the enzyme SAMe synthetase and thus SAMe production, it makes sense that administering SAMe would simply bypass the production step and the process would continue.

SAMe is the product of combining the amino acid methionine and adenosine tri-phosphate (ATP), the body's "energy molecule." This process requires an enzyme called

S-adenomethionine synthetase (or SAMe synthetase). Cirrhosis seems to cause a great deal of damage to SAMe synthetase, so that methionine does not get converted to SAMe. This has two major effects. First, the body retains a higher level of methionine, which can cause poisoning problems in itself. Second, and most important, the liver is unable to make bile salts, which decreases its ability to make bile, which in turn decreases the body's ability to digest fats.

Since cirrhosis appears to inhibit the enzyme SAMe synthetase[1] and thus SAMe production, it makes sense that administering SAMe would simply bypass the production step and the process would continue. The exogenous SAMe would donate the methyl groups needed to make bile salts, so the liver could manufacture bile, which would be used to digest fats, and so on. And it appears that this is exactly what happens.

The Evidence

Several studies seem to show that giving SAMe to persons with cirrhotic livers results in an increase in the taurine aspects of bile salts, thus restoring the bile function. In one study, 10 patients with cirrhosis received 800 mg orally of SAMe a day for two months. Bile samples showed an increase in gluthamic acid as well as an increase in the bile salts that included taurine.[2]

Another study also noted an increase in glutathione and taurine in patients with liver disease after administration of SAMe. The researchers particularly noted that cirrhotic patients were at increased risk for liver damage from substances that are normally detoxified by glutathione. The administration of SAMe reduced the toxicity in the liver by increasing the glutathione concentration.[3]

Another researcher specifically studied the decrease in the enzyme SAMe synthetase in 26 patients with cirrhosis, 12 from alcohol and 14 from post-hepatic blockage. This study noted a marked deficiency in SAMe as a result of the deficiency of SAMe synthetase.[4] Yet another researcher noticed particularly that prolonged alcohol ingestion inhibited SAMe synthetase.[5]

Four studies, three of which were double-blind, observed the results of administering SAMe over a period of time. One double-blind study evaluated 20 patients with hepatic cirrhosis from various causes, including alcohol. The patients received 30 mg of SAMe in six oral doses a day, along with vitamin B12. The researchers measured various liver functions. These included protein production, specifically albumin; the ability of the liver to metabolize bilirubin, which is a breakdown of red blood cell products; and its ability to diffuse immune molecules. After 30 days of therapy, all of these functions showed improvement. A control group of 20 patients received B12 alone in the same doses; these patients showed no improvement in the parameters that improved in the SAMe patients.[6]

Another double-blind study measured the activity of SAMe in hepatic cirrhosis. Twenty-eight patients received 150 mg IV of SAMe daily, plus 2,000 units of vitamin B12. The control group of 25 patients received B12 alone. The SAMe group showed significant improvement in hepatic function, including a return to normal protein synthesis.[7]

A similar study was conducted with 70 hospitalized patients who had chronic hepatitis that was either persistent or aggressive, and who therefore showed varying severity of hepatic cirrhosis. One group was treated with 15 mg IV of SAMe twice a day for 20 days. The other group received 20 mg IV of a fructose salt, with molecules that are similar in size to SAMe.

This study specifically measured protein production, particularly albumin. Protein production returned to normal in patients who received SAMe.[8]

Finally, a double-blind study attempted a similar experiment, giving 15 cirrhotic patients 15 mg doses of SAMe four times a day, either IM or IV, for 30 days. Another 15 patients received l-methionine and ATP, the precursors to SAMe. The measure was to see if albumin production improved or returned to normal. It did return to normal function in the SAMe-treated group, while the other group showed no improvement. Not only did this prove that the therapeutic effects were due to SAMe, it also increased the probability that the problem in cirrhosis is SAMe synthetase.[9]

With SAMe, there's a good chance that the liver of a person with cirrhosis, while not regenerating completely, may improve enough to enable the person to lead a longer, healthier life.

Another study was based on the knowledge that alcohol reduces the pool of glutathione in the mitochondria by preventing the transport of glutathione into the mitochondria.

The researchers were able to demonstrate that the introduction of SAMe actually improved that transport.[10] This is a particularly interesting concept, because what we are actually seeing is the ability of SAMe to improve the flow through membranes. Improved flow across cell membranes in the brain may be a factor in SAMe's beneficial effects on depression. We also have evidence that SAMe improves flow through the membranes of erythrocytes (red blood cells)[11] and increases the flow of fluids into cartilage. This is probably one of the reasons that SAMe is considered to be chondroprotective; that is, it has the ability to protect cartilage as well as increasing its function and building it up.

To test this concept, another group of researchers measured the concentration of the sulfurated products that come out of SAMe mediation, particularly glutathione and cysteine. They did this by checking the concentrations of these substances in erythrocytes in 20 alcohol misusers with cirrhosis and 20 subjects without it. Both groups received 2 grams IV of SAMe daily. Concentrations of glutathione and cysteine improved in both groups. Since these substances are necessary for the production and proper functioning of red blood cells, this experiment suggests that SAMe is actually somewhat protective even in active alcoholics, although it is not as protective as stopping drinking.[12]

All of this indicates that SAMe attacks cirrhosis of the liver on all fronts. It increases the ability of the mitochondria to accept substances. It increases the ability of the liver to regenerate itself. And it improves the liver's ability to make protein and metabolize substances. In short, SAMe seems to help the liver go back to doing its job. With SAMe, there's a good chance that the liver of a person with cirrhosis, while not regenerating completely, may improve enough to enable the person to lead a longer, healthier life.

Of course, all this is theoretical, because thus far there are no long-term studies to bear it out. The evidence certainly warrants conducting such studies, and I hope this book plays a part in stimulating such research.

CHAPTER 11

SAMe AND FIBROMYALGIA

As I said in the introduction, despite its benefits, SAMe is not a cure-all, or even a cure-most. We have seen clear evidence for its usefulness in treating osteoarthritis, depression, and liver disease. In the next couple of chapters we'll look at conditions that SAMe is purported to help, but for which the evidence is much less definitive. These include fibromyalgia, Parkinson's disease, and Alzheimer's disease.

What Is Fibromyalgia?

Fibromyalgia is a mysterious and frustrating chronic ailment that affects about 2 percent of the population—some six million Americans. Two-thirds of fibromyalgia sufferers are women.[1] Fibromyalgia is most commonly seen in people between the ages of 30 and 60,[2] and it is the third or fourth most prevalent condition that rheumatologists see.[3]

The chief features of fibromyalgia are widespread pain, sleep disturbances, and overwhelming fatigue, but it can also include a broad range of other symptoms:

- Morning stiffness

- Gastrointestinal problems

- Headaches

- Paresthesia (numbness or tingling)

- Cystitis (bladder pain)

- Vision problems

- Allergic symptoms

- Chronic vaginal yeast infections in women

- Mental "fogginess"

- Mood disorders, including depression

A significant minority of patients complain of chemical sensitivities as well. Many people are partially to completely disabled by their symptoms; an estimated 25 percent of patients seen in rheumatology clinics have received disability payments for fibromyalgia.[4] For many patients, the relentless fatigue and the inability to get restful sleep are more disabling than the pain.

Because it is characterized by musculoskeletal pain, fibromyalgia has been classified as a rheumatological disorder, and it has even been called a type of arthritis. However, studies of the muscles of fibromyalgia patients, using electromyography (EMG) and biopsies of the painful tissue have not turned up any evidence of muscle pathology or inflammation. Fibromyalgia pain is not necessarily the result of overstressed muscles such as one might find in tension headaches. Despite efforts to find one, there are as yet no objective laboratory markers for fibromyalgia; it is diagnosed on the basis of symptoms and the presence of "tender points," that is, specific locations on the body that create moderate to severe pain when pressed.

Considerable crossover of symptoms exists among fibromyalgia, myofascial pain syndrome, chronic fatigue syndrome, and the illness dubbed Gulf War syndrome. Some researchers believe all these conditions are manifestations of the same disorder, or at least that they are somehow related. Unlike diseases such as osteoarthritis, heart disease, or cancer, these illnesses have no abnormalities that can be traced to a specific, identifiable cause or location in the brain or body. This makes them immensely frustrating for both patients and doctors, most of whom would prefer a clear-cut problem that they can address with a specific treatment, rather than a diffuse collection of symptoms that seem to have no unifying factor or cause.

A System-Wide Disorder

Evidence indicates that fibromyalgia is actually a systemic disorder involving the central nervous system, the endocrine system, and possibly the immune system as well. I should point out that separating these functions into different systems is somewhat misleading, as they are all interconnected and interdependent. It might be better to call fibromyalgia a disorder of the neuroendocrine-immune system. A number of studies have looked at fibromyalgia as a dysfunction of the limbic system, in particular the hypothalamus.[5-14] These studies suggest that fibromyalgia's diverse symptoms result from disturbances in the brain's ability to properly regulate many body functions including:

- Hormone production and distribution,

- Temperature regulation

- The sleep-wake cycle

- Various metabolic functions

- The autonomic nervous system

- And even blood flow to the brain

One primary aspect of fibromyalgia is the inability of a person to achieve level four, or deep sleep. This is the stage of sleep during which our brains produce serotonin and growth hormone, which is needed for muscle repair. Studies in which normal subjects were deprived of stage four sleep for a period of several days found that they developed fibromyalgia-like symptoms. Thus, some researchers regard fibromyalgia as primarily a sleep disorder, although this may be a chicken-and-egg type situation—the pain prevents deep sleep, which leads to pain, and so on.

Is It Really Depression?

Because fibromyalgia shows a lack of identifiable abnormalities combined with a high level of responses from the central nervous system, a number of researchers have attempted to make the association between fibromyalgia and depression, even suggesting that fibromyalgia may be a variant of depression. This has led to a certain defensiveness among many fibromyalgia patients, who see it as a dismissal and an invalidation of their suffering. Part of the problem stems from western medicine's insistence on separating disease into two categories—mental (or emotional) and physical—with the latter category somehow being more real, or at least easier to deal with. To be categorized as a physical disease, a condition must have some objective marker—such as a swollen, deformed joint or a colony of cancer cells—that can be detected with the naked eye or through the assistance of some machine or laboratory test. In this view, since fibromyalgia has no such marker, it must be a psychological condition. To me, this entire argument begs the question, since the mind and body are not separate entities but interconnected parts of a unified whole. Therefore, all illness is physical, mental, *and* emotional to some extent, and the boundaries between those aspects are pretty blurry.

Fibromyalgia is a mysterious and frustrating chronic ailment that affects about 2 percent of the population—some six million Americans.

That being said, let's look at the evidence for and against fibromyalgia being a form of depression. To begin with, the symptoms of depression and fibromyalgia are often similar, as are the associated disorders such as headaches, irritable bowel syndrome, and sleep disturbances. Also, a large number of patients with fibromyalgia have relatives who suffer from depression, and many patients with fibromyalgia suffer from depression themselves. In addition, one of the few pharmacological treatments for fibromyalgia that has shown any success is the use of antidepressant medications, although the benefits are often temporary. These factors, along with the lack of diagnostic tests that can distinguish fibromyalgia from other disease processes such as depression, have led a number of researchers to postulate a relationship between the two conditions.[15]

The mainstay for the pharmacological treatment of fibromyalgia lies in controlling pain and treating the underlying sleep disorder.

However, the studies making the relationship between fibromyalgia and depression are not uniform, and they are often not very good. Further, although the conditions demonstrate some common characteristics, they also have some marked differences. For example, antidepressants may be somewhat helpful in treating fibromyalgia, but they are not the only treatment or necessarily the most appropriate one. In addition, the dosages of tricyclics used to treat fibromyalgia are much lower than those used for major depressive disorders.

Many of the studies on the use of antidepressants for fibromyalgia did not show a close correlation between improvement in the psychological symptoms and the physical symptoms.[16] All of this is borne out by indications that SAMe is helpful for depression, but does not appear to be of much benefit in treating fibromyalgia, as we shall see.

Thus, current evidence does not demonstrate a close enough relationship between fibromyalgia and depression to state that they are the same condition, although in my opinion the issue warrants further investigation. It is also important to recognize that the depression associated with fibromyalgia could as much be an effect of the pain and fatigue as a cause of them.

Treatments for Fibromyalgia

The four major components of a fibromyalgia treatment program are: the use of drugs to control pain and aid sleep, exercise to reduce pain and increase mobility, education and support for what the patient is dealing with, and stress reduction.

Pharmacological Treatments

The mainstay for the pharmacological treatment of fibromyalgia lies in controlling pain and treating the underlying sleep disorder. Unfortunately, no medication has been found to be wholly effective for fibromyalgia pain, and doctors and patients may have to cooperate in finding something that works at least moderately well. Some people have success with anti-inflammatories; others get relief with muscle relaxants such as Flexeril, Robaxin, or Parafon Forte, or with synthetic opiates such as Ultram.

Studies have shown the tricyclic antidepressants to be most valuable, providing some pain relief and particularly helping to improve sleep. As I stated earlier, the doses used for fibromyalgia, as well as for chronic fatigue syndrome, are considerably lower than those normally used in major depression. The standard dose of amitriptyline for fibromyalgia is 25 to 75 mg per day, versus 150 to 300 mg per day for depression.[17] Unfortunately, many people cannot tolerate the side effects of the tricyclics, and they stop taking the medication.

Low levels of the neurotransmitter serotonin are associated with both depression and fibromyalgia. The brain metabolism of depression also appears to involve norepinephrine, a catecholamine. Interestingly, those antidepressant drugs that relate more closely to serotonin uptake appear to be more effective in alleviating fibromyalgia pain, while those that deal more with the catecholamines (neurotransmitters that cause excitatory responses in the brain and body) are more effective in dealing with depressive symptoms.

In the realm of alternative medications, valerian root, tryptophan, and 5-HTP, all of which are used to relieve anxiety and stress symptoms, are reported to be helpful in fibromyalgia as well.

Exercise

Exercise is an essential component of any fibromyalgia treatment program.[18–21] I can't emphasize this enough. Just as with any musculoskeletal or rheumatological disease, if you succumb to the pain and limit your activity, the pain will get worse until even small movements become painful. The only thing accomplished by reducing your activity is to increase the amount of pain you feel at lower and lower activity levels—a serious consequence indeed.

Therefore, a regular exercise program that involves both aerobic and stretching activities is not only encouraged, but universally accepted as mandatory for reducing fibromyalgia pain. This works two ways:

1. Muscles that are stretched and moved regularly stay looser and are less painful to move. If you keep even a healthy muscle contracted for a long time, it will hurt when you try to stretch it—a fact known to anyone who has ever been in a cast. When a joint or limb is immobilized for any length of time, the ligaments contract and the muscles get weaker, so that initial attempts at movement cause considerable discomfort.

2. Moving the muscle makes it stronger, and the stronger a muscle is, the more stress and activity it can handle.

Some people go so far as to say that the goal of exercise for fibromyalgia patients is not to eradicate pain, but to increase mobility. I would suggest by increasing mobility one actually does decrease pain, maybe not completely, but certainly relative to someone who restricts movement. Forms of aerobic exercise that are good for fibromyalgia patients include low impact aerobics, water aerobics, and walking. Swimming is an excellent form of exercise because it involves the whole body. Yoga, which involves a series of gentle stretches, is also excellent for improving a person's flexibility and strength, as well as for reducing stress, which in itself helps relieve pain.

As with arthritis, some people may need biomechanics instruction to discover ways they are holding and moving their bodies that may be increasing their pain, and to help change those patterns. Additionally, many people find massage to be helpful for relieving pain and reducing stress. It is important to have a massage therapist who understands and is experienced at working with fibromyalgia patients, as overaggressive massage can actually make the pain worse.

Education and Support

A major part of the work I do with fibromyalgia patients involves educating them about the processes involved in fibromyalgia, what we know about it, what works (and what doesn't), and what they can expect. This goes a long way toward relieving their feelings of helplessness and frustration. I also offer support and validation—the most important validation being that the person has pain. Many people with fibromyalgia are understandably resentful when doctors or others refuse to believe that they are in pain because "nothing shows up on any tests." The pain of fibromyalgia is undeniably real, and patients deserve to have that recognized.

If all a healer does is validate a patient's pain, however, he will have little success in helping the patient overcome the the disease. Working with people who have fibromyalgia requires a great deal of tact and skill, because they tend to be as sensitive emotionally as they are physically. Nevertheless, going beyond the surface symptoms can uncover important patterns that can help a person begin to heal.

What I am about to say is anecdotal, based on my own experience, but I believe it is valid nonetheless. It has become something of a truism that different personality factors make people susceptible to certain illnesses. For example, links have been observed between hostility and heart disease; a tendency to repress emotions and cancer; and, as I discussed earlier, internal conflicts and depression. This is not to say that people cause their illnesses or are to blame for them, only that we all have different susceptibilities. What I have observed in fibromyalgia patients are certain emotional patterns related to hyperalertness, a need for protection, and a feeling of extreme vulnerability to the people and elements around them. I also find images of isolation, a belief that they are not being supported, and a lack of the skills to live successfully in a world they perceive as hostile. None of these elements and perceptions are without basis. The problem lies with the emphasis on the world's hostility and the vulnerability that a person feels in it, as well as a lack of balance in seeing other aspects of the world. Interestingly, a common thread among many fibromyalgia patients is a history of physical, emotional, or sexual abuse, which could certainly account for feeling vulnerable in a dangerous and hostile world.

. . . a regular exercise program that involves both aerobic and stretching activities is not only encouraged, but universally accepted as mandatory for reducing fibromyalgia pain.

If patients are willing to look at these factors, they can make considerable progress in getting better. I find such willingness surprisingly common once my patients realize my desire is to help them rather than to assign an emotional cause to their illness. I try to offer all of my patients, not just those with fibromyalgia, a firm sense of support. My goal is to give them the courage to test reality, that is, to consider a different interpretation of their perceptions of reality and to examine how those perceptions may affect their behavior and health. As the supportive relationship develops, this reality testing becomes more legitimate, valid, and helpful to the patient.

Stress Reduction

I have already discussed the role of stress in causing and aggravating many disease processes. This is true times ten for fibromyalgia. Many sufferers date the beginning of their symptoms to an episode of extreme physical and/or psychological stress, and virtually all report that stress triggers or worsens their symptoms. Since this is so, learning to manage stress is a major help in alleviating those symptoms.

At its most basic, stress reduction consists of learning and using techniques such as progressive muscle relaxation, guided imagery, and meditation. These techniques are most effective when the patient does them consistently, at or about the same time each day. Turning them into a ritual causes an unconscious body reaction, a responsive relaxation in expectation of the event to come.

By paying attention to your emotions and your body, you can learn to associate particular emotional events with painful muscular episodes. Knowing what triggers attacks can make it easier for you to head them off, such as by changing a stressful situation—or changing your response to it. This is admittedly difficult, but becomes easier with practice. Psychotherapy, particularly the behavioral and cognitive forms, can be useful for learning these types of emotional skills.

SAMe and Fibromyalgia

As I stated earlier, part of the evidence that fibromyalgia and depression are different disorders is the fact that SAMe does not seem to be all that effective at relieving fibromyalgia symptoms. One double-blind study compared SAMe with a placebo. The study included 44 patients who received 800 mg of SAMe or a placebo each day for six weeks. Results were measured using the FACE scale and the Beck depression inventory, two evaluative processes. Although the SAMe group showed significantly more improvement than the placebo group with respect to pain, fatigue, morning stiffness, and mood, as evaluated by the FACE scale, researchers found no difference between groups with respect to sensitivity at tender points, muscle strength, and mood as evaluated by the Beck depression inventory. Both groups experienced similar side effects.[22]

Another double-blind study involved 34 patients who received 600 mg of either SAMe or a placebo intravenously over ten days. The SAMe group showed a slightly higher statistical improvement for subjective pain at rest, pain in movement, and overall well-being, as well as improvement in sleep, fatigue, and morning stiffness. Again, however, there was no difference in tender point sensitivity or muscle strength between the two groups.[23]

A third double-blind study comparing SAMe with a placebo evaluated 17 patients with primary fibromyalgia. Eleven had significant depression as assessed by HAM-D or an

Italian depression-rating scale called Scala di Autovalutazione per la Depressione (SAD). Both depression and trigger-point pain improved after SAMe administration but not after the placebo.[24]

Thus it would appear that the use of SAMe for fibromyalgia . . . does not seem to hold the obvious promise that we found with other conditions, except that it relieves the depressive symptoms . . . However, . . . the fact that patients reported subjective improvement in their symptoms warrants further research.

How do we account for these results? One explanation is that SAMe brought about improvement in patients' moods, which made their fibromyalgia symptoms less troubling. Thus, it would appear that the use of SAMe for fibromyalgia, albeit incompletely studied at this point, does not seem to hold the obvious promise that we found with other conditions, except that it relieves the depressive symptoms that often accompany the disease. However, the existing studies were small and short-term, and the fact that patients reported subjective improvement in their symptoms warrants further research. Perhaps in a future edition of this book I will have better, or at least more conclusive, news for fibromyalgia sufferers.

CHAPTER 12

SAMe, PARKINSON'S DISEASE, AND ALZHEIMER'S DISEASE

One of the dangers in interpreting any kind of scientific research is mistaking association for cause and effect. An association simply means that a mutual relationship exists between two or more things or conditions. For example, low levels of serotonin are found in a number of conditions, including depression, fibromyalgia, and Parkinson's disease (PD). Thus, there is an association between low serotonin levels and those conditions. This does not mean, however, that a lack of serotonin causes the conditions, any more than a pitcher's refusal to change his socks during a winning streak causes him to throw strikes. Nor does it necessarily mean that artificially boosting serotonin levels will cause the condition to improve.

The association/cause-and-effect error is one of the fallacies behind many supplement fads today (as well as many assertions in conventional research). For example, people's bodies tend to manufacture less of the hormone DHEA as they age. Thus, there is an association (albeit an imperfect one) between aging and a decreased level of DHEA. Identifying this relationship led to speculation that raising DHEA levels could stop or reverse the aging process—speculation that quickly turned into a media-fueled stampede to get in on the latest anti-aging miracle.

Alas, it's just not that simple. Our bodies are elaborate chemical factories, operating at a level of complexity that all of our best science has yet to explain or comprehend. Attempting to micromanage this process, based on our limited knowledge, is at best a gamble. Sometimes we win, and people get better. Other times our attempts have no effect at all, and sometimes we even make things worse.

Researchers have identified associations between low levels of SAMe and a number of different conditions, including osteoarthritis and liver disease. In those cases, we saw that augmenting SAMe actually does bring about improvement in the condition. Now we are going to look at a pair of instances where raising low SAMe levels does not necessarily help and may actually make the condition worse: Parkinson's disease and Alzheimer's disease.

Parkinson's Disease

Parkinson's disease is a degenerative disease of an area of the mid-brain called the substantia nigra. The substantia nigra contains pigmented neurons that manufacture dopamine, a neurotransmitter that is critical to motor function. In Parkinson's disease, the substantia nigra breaks down, and the pigmented neurons begin to die off. Just as you can lose up to 80 percent of your liver or kidneys and still function reasonably well, you can lose up to 80 percent of these neurons before you start to show symptoms of Parkinson's disease. Thus, doctors tend to see Parkinson's disease only in its advanced stages, which means it is usually diagnosed in people in their fifties and sixties. It affects more men than women, by a three to two ratio.

One of the dangers in interpreting any kind of scientific research is mistaking association for cause and effect.

In recent years, researchers have learned a great deal about Parkinson's disease, thanks to a California designer drug called methylphenyltetrahydropyridine (MPTP), which has allowed them to study the disorder extensively in animals. However, the causes of the disease are still not known, although some epidemiologists have suggested that industrial toxins may play a part. As much as I emphasize the need to exercise, eat a good diet, and avoid putting a lot of toxins in your body, I cannot associate the failure to do any of these with Parkinson's. There seems to be no behavioral reason why a person develops Parkinson's disease.

Signs and Symptoms

Parkinson's disease can be thought of as a general, inexorable slowing down of the brain and body. The hallmark of the disease is a pattern of disturbed movement. People with Parkinson's disease suffer a simultaneous decrease in their ability to start or stop voluntary movements (such as walking), and an increase in involuntary movements. These include characteristic tremors, such as a shaking hand that may be accompanied by a twisting of the wrist. A particular feature of the disease is a movement called pill-rolling, where the thumb and the forefinger or the middle finger move back and forth against each other, as if the patient were rolling a pill out of clay. Parkinson's sufferers usually have a stooped posture, and their gait is slow and shuffling. In addition, their handwriting gets slower and smaller (micrographia), and their speech becomes slower and decreases in volume. The slowness of movement is called bradykinesia.

Parkinson's disease can be thought of as a general, inexorable slowing down of the brain and body. The hallmark of the disease is a pattern of disturbed movement.

The bodies of persons with PD are rigid and appear tensed up and wooden. They also exhibit a trait called cogwheeling; if you were to grasp a Parkinson patient's flexed arm and attempt to pull it out, it would straighten in jerky steps, as if it were a lever connected to a cogwheel. This muscular rigidity leads to a lot of muscle and back pain. Other symptoms include sleep disturbances and sexual dysfunction.

The behavioral changes that accompany Parkinson's disease include apathy, decreased confidence, fearfulness, and anxiety, all of which could be considered secondary effects of the inability to move around. A person's thought processes are significantly slower. Parkinson's patients can actually be somewhat demented, and in serious cases may suffer from disorientation, paranoia, hallucinations, and occasionally psychosis, although this is not common. Depression is common among Parkinson's patients, but this is most likely a response to the devastating effects of the disease itself, rather than a direct consequence of Parkinson's effects on the brain.

Conventional Treatment for Parkinson's Disease

Currently, the chief treatment for Parkinson's disease consists of bolstering the body's dwindling ability to make dopamine. This is accomplished by loading the system with dopamine's precursor, an amino acid called dihydroxyphenylalanine (DOPA). Generally, two drugs, levodopa (or L-dopa) and carbidopa, are used in combination with one another. Less frequently, dopamine agonists, or enhancers, such as bromocriptine and pergolide are used in tandem with the L-dopa combination. At first, these drugs are generally effective in reducing the signs and symptoms of the disease. Unfortunately, they do not stop the underlying degeneration. Over time, the dosage must be increased, and eventually the patient stops responding to the drugs altogether.

In the past, anticholinergics (drugs that block the action the neurotransmitter acetylcholine) such as trihexylphenadol and benztropine were used to treat Parkinson's disease, but L-dopa is so much more effective that these have become second line drugs. Other drugs that have been used include amantadine, an anti-viral agent that has demonstrated some anti-Parkinson effects; and deprenyl, an MAO inhibitor that is used mainly for depression. Inhibiting the MAO increases norepinephrine levels, which seems to help motor activity as well as depression. As you may recall from Chapter 8, MAO inhibitors carry significant risks, particularly with regard to their interaction with certain foods.

L-dopa generally has few side effects. Too high a dose can cause hallucinations, and some patients experience vivid dreams. In rare cases it can cause psychosis. Other effects include nausea, vomiting, postural hypotension (a drop in blood pressure upon standing), and very rarely, cardiac arrhythmia. Most of these effects are dose-related. Adding carbidopa enhances L-dopa's effectiveness and reduces the need for high doses, thus lowering the possibility of adverse effects.

Other Treatments

In the past decade, researchers have explored a number of experimental treatments for Parkinson's disease. One of the best known and more controversial approaches involves implanting brain cells from the substantia nigra of fetuses into the brains of Parkinson's patients. A more recent development involves transplanting cloned animal brain cells that secrete dopamine. Although still being investigated, this latter technique has shown some promise, and it could be clinically available within this decade.

Finally, as with most other chronic or degenerative diseases, the most important treatment for Parkinson's disease is keeping active. Regular physical exercise, especially stretching, can be of great benefit to Parkinson's patients. Yoga, particularly hatha yoga, is one way to keep the body limber and flexible, thus minimizing the devastating muscular effects of the disease. Emotional and social support are critical, along with increasing physical support as the person becomes more and more debilitated. As with other illnesses, the symptoms of PD are aggravated by stress. Therefore, reducing stress helps reduce the frequency and severity of symptoms.

SAMe and Parkinson's Disease

At least one study has shown that persons with Parkinson's disease have significantly lower levels of SAMe than normal control subjects. In fact, the normal subjects had almost twice as much SAMe as the Parkinson's patients. However, it is possible that this is part of a compensatory strategy by the body. Increased methylation decreases the levels of dopamine, norepinephrine, and a substance called 5 hydroxytriptamine, or 5HT. At the same time, methylation increases acetylcholine, a neurotransmitter that plays a part in telling the muscles to contract, among other functions. These changes cause the same impaired movement (called hypokinesia) and tremors that are hallmarks of Parkinson's disease. Since SAMe is a methyl donor, perhaps the body is lowering SAMe levels in order to slow methylation and counteract the effects of PD.

Earlier, I mentioned a study in which SAMe was injected into the lateral ventricle of the brains of rats. The rats in that study demonstrated the signs of Parkinson's disease: tremors, rigidity, hypokinesia, and depleted dopamine.[1] In a different study in which SAMe was injected into the lateral ventricle of the brains of rats, the rats showed decreased motor activity.[2]

These studies seem to support the idea that the brain can have too much SAMe. However, another study found that treatment with the methyl donors betaine, methionine, and SAMe helped improve depression and cognitive function in patients with dementia—but these patients did not have PD.

Currently, the chief treatment for Parkinson's disease consists of bolstering the body's dwindling ability to make dopamine.

In summary, the evidence suggests that L-dopa depletes SAMe, and that the presence of high levels of SAMe in the brain can lead to high methylation, which is detrimental to controlling symptoms in Parkinson's disease. This leads me to believe that we should be careful about using SAMe in Parkinson's patients, even if it is only to treat the depression that often accompanies this devastating disease.

Alzheimer's Disease

Alzheimer's disease is a devastating, progressive dementia that is quite common in the elderly and becomes more common as a person ages. It is characterized by decreased amounts of neurotransmitters in the brain. However, attempts to increase the amount of neurotransmitters do not appear to either slow the disease's progress or improve its symptoms, and none of the various drugs on the market have turned out to be as effective as initially hoped.

Like Parkinson's disease, Alzheimer's appears to have many connections with SAMe. Whether these relationships are merely associative, or administering SAMe would have some actual benefits, is open to exploration.

Symptoms and Effects

The symptoms of Alzheimer's disease are gradually progressive, consisting of diminishing capacity in three areas:

1. Decreased ability to remember, especially short-term memory

2. Spatial difficulties

3. Inability to remember names of persons or things, called anomic aphasia

People with Alzheimer's disease frequently act in inappropriate or even bizarre ways: neglecting personal hygiene; walking into public areas unsuitably clothed or with no clothes; exhibiting a course, crude sense of humor; wandering; and displaying outbursts of temper (sometimes called a catastrophic reaction). As the disease advances, patients may show greater rigidity in their arms and legs and often have difficulty initiating walking. Seizures can occur very late in the course of Alzheimer's disease.

No tests currently exist for diagnosing Alzheimer's disease, and the diagnosis is often made by observing the progressive symptoms. CT scans and MRI can show widespread atrophy, which is suggestive of the disease. It's important to remember that not all dementia is Alzheimer's disease, and dementia may be due to a number of different, treatable causes. These include depression, B12 deficiency, drug effects, or chronic infections.

SAMe and Alzheimer's Disease

The relationship between SAMe and Alzheimer's disease has yet to be examined in depth. However, some evidence suggests SAMe's role with respect to particular cells and activities that may be involved in Alzheimer's disease.

Several studies have looked at the concentrations of SAMe during different stages of development and aging in both animals and humans. These studies show that SAMe levels are high at the beginning of life and decrease with age. For example, one study found high concentrations of SAMe in the lenses of day-old rats. The levels gradually declined as the rats got older.[3] On the other end of the spectrum, SAMe is decreased by as much as 25 percent in old rats.[4] This decrease does not seem to relate to nutritional deficiencies such as a lack of folate, but appears to be connected to aging itself.[5] Another study found that SAMe concentrations in humans decreased between infancy and childhood, declining sharply during the first year of life.[6]

Autopsies of older adults with Alzheimer's disease show decreased levels of SAMe in the brain. A decreased level of SAMe was not found in autopsies of persons with Parkinson's disease. This suggests that decreased levels of SAMe are not related to degeneration of the brain due to chronic disease.[7] All of this seems to imply either diminished production or gradually increased utilization of SAMe from birth throughout life. Other research supports the suggestion that the reason SAMe concentrations decrease with age is not because it is being produced at a lesser rate, but because it is being utilized much more rapidly.[8]

Regular physical exercise, especially stretching, can be of great benefit to Parkinson's patients.

Other studies that may have some significance in Alzheimer's disease relate to SAMe's ability to increase the permeability of cell membranes. As we saw in Chapter 10, this is a significant benefit in cirrhosis of the liver, and it may relate to SAMe's effectiveness in depression and osteoarthritis as well. Perhaps it also applies to older brain cells (not necessarily the brain cells of older persons; contrary to popular belief, the brain continues to make new cells throughout life). Levels of certain receptors in the brain are lower in aging animals as compared to younger ones, and SAMe has been shown to increase the density of these receptors. One researcher has theorized that this relates to increased phospholipid synthesis, an important function in brain metabolism.[9,10] Interestingly enough, SAMe does not appear to have any restorative effect on dopamine receptors, which may indicate why it does not appear to benefit Parkinson's disease patients.[11] Furthermore, SAMe showed a disappointingly minimal ability to support myelin, an element in nerve lining.[12]

Thus far, no clinical experiments have studied the effects of SAMe on Alzheimer's disease. However, it may be a promising area to explore, as it is likely that at least some of the disease's effects are due to decreased permeability of cell membranes, which in turn keeps neurotransmitters from getting to their necessary receptors. Because the development of Alzheimer's disease is such a slow process, any study would have to last a significant period of time, at least six months to a year, to be valid.

Thus far, no clinical experiments have studied the effects of SAMe on Alzheimer's disease. However, it may be a promising area to explore . . .

In summary, although the neurodegenerative diseases certainly show some relationship with SAMe processes in the body, the research, especially in the clinical arena, is far short of showing any benefits from SAMe supplementation. I would hope, however, that researchers will be motivated to give SAMe a closer look, especially with regard to Alzheimer's disease.

CHAPTER 13

WORKING
WITH YOUR DOCTOR

Because SAMe is a supplement rather than a drug, and available through retail or mail order outlets, you do not need a doctor to prescribe it. In fact, you need not involve a doctor at all. If you have, or think you have, a condition that SAMe might help, and you can afford to buy it, there is nothing to prevent you from taking it, with or without a doctor's okay. You may perceive this accessibility as being one of the main advantages of supplements over prescription drugs. I'd like you to examine this supposition more closely, however, because easy access may not be as clear an advantage as it seems to be. I'd also like you to examine your relationship with your doctor, assuming you have one (if you don't, think about why not) and consider the following questions:

- Do you regard your doctor as an ally or an adversary?

- Do you consider him a knowledgeable professional or simply an overpaid technician?

- Is your relationship one of mutual respect, mutual resentment, or perhaps worse, mutual indifference?

These are important questions, which rarely get asked. What I'm trying to get at here is that the doctor-patient relationship, like any human relationship, goes both ways. We hear a lot these days about deteriorating "quality of care," and there is no doubt that we in the medical profession bear a large share of the responsibility for this perceived decline. But patients must bear some of the blame as well. In this chapter, I'll talk about how you can help make your relationship with your doctor a constructive one, based on shared responsibility and cooperation and dedicated to one key objective—improving and maintaining your health.

Why You Should Have a Doctor As Your Health Care Partner

Certainly you don't always need a physician to determine the appropriate treatment for a health-related problem. For example, if you have a headache, your own knowledge and experience may tell you that aspirin, acetaminophen, or ibuprofen will be an effective remedy, or at least the first thing to try. If you have a cold, taking a decongestant and a cough reliever, along with lots of fluids and some rest, are effective treatments that don't require any medical intervention. In the same way, if you are suffering from osteoarthritis (and know for a fact that it is OA), taking SAMe at the recommended doses for a period of a few weeks will demonstrate whether it will work for you or not, without the help of any expert.

Working in partnership with a good doctor can help you gain a greater sense of how your body works and how you can best take care of it.

Sometimes, however, you need a second opinion, preferably one backed by knowledge and experience. For example, a sudden, severe headache may be a symptom of a stroke, while chronic headaches can indicate anything from the need for a new eyeglass prescription to a brain tumor. And what if that joint pain is not osteoarthritis at all, but something else that SAMe (or glucosamine) won't help and another treatment could help?

Working in partnership with a good doctor can help you gain a greater sense of how your body works and how you can take the best possible care of it. You can learn how to handle minor ailments appropriately, and how to judge when an office visit or phone call to your doctor is actually warranted. You can get help for managing a chronic condition so you can lead a full life in spite of it. You can protect yourself from potential errors—such as combining potent herbs and prescription drugs—that could put you in danger. In short, a doctor whom you respect, and who respects you, can be your strongest ally in protecting that most valuable of possessions—your health.

The Nature of the Patient-Doctor Relationship

Philosopher Martin Buber identified two key types of relationships. One is an I-it relationship, in which a person ("I") acts upon an object ("it"). The "it" can be either a person or a thing. The actor's purpose is to manipulate the object to meet a need or desire, and the object's purpose is to fulfill a specific function or functions required by the actor. An example of an I-it relationship is that of a driver to a street. The street exists merely to drive upon, and the driver neither wants nor needs anything else from it. The relationship is simple and profitable for both parties, although the profit for the street is solely one of existence. The street's responsibility, if it can be called that, is simply to fulfill its function, which is maintaining a flat, relatively even surface on which to travel. When it ceases to perform this function, it ceases to contribute appropriately to the relationship. The driver's responsibility to the street is negligible, except perhaps to pay taxes for its maintenance.

The other type of relationship is I-thou, in which reciprocity is not only expected, but demanded. An I-thou relationship offers benefits to both participants, and both have a responsibility to the relationship. I-thou relationships can exist only between conscious entities. Usually this means people, although it is also possible to have I-thou relationships, as well as I-it ones, between people and animals (whether I-thou relationships can exist between animals is a subject for another book).

Just because an I-thou relationship requires consciousness does not mean that all relationships between conscious beings are I-thou. We all have many relationships in which, although we talk to people and hear or see some response, neither party has any desire for interaction beyond meeting an immediate need. Take, for example, shopping. When you go to a store, you collect items and bring them to a clerk, whose function is to scan or enter them into the cash register, ask for money, hand you the proper change (or a charge slip to sign), and bag the items for you to take away. For you, this is the epitome of an I-it relationship. But it is also an I-it relationship for the clerk, who sees your function as bringing the items to the cash register in the proper way, handing over sufficient funds to pay for them, and taking them away when the transaction is complete. You speak and listen to one another, you may even smile, say "please" and "thank you," and exchange pleasantries (or irritations), but in the vast majority of cases, the relationship goes no deeper.

Unfortunately, too many of our relationships are of the I-it variety, including those that by their very nature should be much more meaningful. The fact that so many marriages end in divorce could, in part, reflect a tendency to treat this most fundamental of relationships as I-it; a tendency that has no doubt existed for a very long time. That the divorce rate is higher now than in the past is probably due not so much to a shift in husband-wife relations as to the fact that society has given people permission to leave when they tire of either being treated or treating their spouses as objects. Similarly, we tend to treat many of our professional relationships as I-it, whether we are acting as the client or the service provider. We see our attorney, or our accountant, or our doctor in terms of what we perceive their function to be, rather than as our partners in a relationship that supports a mutual goal.

When I ask myself the questions, "What would I want in a professional? What would I want in a physician?" several things come to mind, such as knowledge, skill, wisdom, kindness, and compassion. But the most important of these and the one that stands far and above any other qualities—is integrity.

I have often heard patients bemoan the disappearance of the old-time doctor. He was like a god, they say, knowledgeable, comforting, and wise. In the same breath they declare that he was available for any need they had, day or night. When I hear this, I can't help but wonder if they are describing a god or a slave. To me, it sounds like the quintessential I-it relationship. Nowhere do I get a sense of that doctor as a person with his own strengths, weaknesses, thoughts, needs, and desires. In truth, a doctor is neither a god nor a slave, but a presumably well-trained professional who has knowledge and experience to contribute to a relationship based on a common goal—the health of the patient.

So the question to think about in evaluating your relationship with your doctor, or in choosing a new doctor, is: What kind of a relationship do you want to have with this person? Do you want an interactive relationship in which the caregiver offers her expertise, experience, knowledge, and integrity in support of both your long-term health and your current need to deal with whatever process you are going through at the moment? If so, you are seeking an I-thou relationship.

If, on the other hand, your interest is in meeting specific needs for specific problems, and you already know how you want to address those problems, you probably want to use your caregiver essentially as a living database and a facilitator who can give you access to the treatment you desire. In this case, what you really want is an I-it relationship.

I'm sure that most people reading this would say, "Of course I want the I-thou relationship. It's much more meaningful and enduring." Before jumping in too quickly, however, understand that the I-thou relationship requires a great deal more responsibility and commitment. It means agreeing to do things that advance your common goal—that is, your own good health. It means being willing to talk openly about your concerns *and* to listen to your caregiver's impressions and ideas about what directions you should take. And it means having the patience and perseverance to work through the inevitable disagreements about those directions. I have a number of patients who, from my perspective, can be very disagreeable indeed! But I've found that such conflicts actually enhance our relationship, because they force me to explain myself in a way that the other person will understand. Often, they force both of us to find creative ways to reach consensus. I become a better doctor, the patient becomes a better and a healthier patient, and our relationship deepens.

I suspect many readers at this point will say, "This is good advice, Dr. Grazi, but I belong to an HMO, and I don't get enough time with my doctor to develop that kind of relationship." I must respond that the belief that people don't get quality care because of a lack of time is erroneous. An encounter need not be a long one to be meaningful, if both people are receptive and prepared to focus on what needs to take place during the meeting. All of us know from experience that it need not take a lot of time to "connect" with someone. You can have an I-thou relationship in a two-minute phone call. If you can't establish a connection with your primary provider in the time you have to meet with him, ask for a different one, and keep asking until you get someone you can connect with. (I'll talk about specific qualities to look for in a healer a little later in the chapter.)

You can also get more out of the time you do have by being prepared with your concerns and questions, and getting as many of the latter answered ahead of time as possible. Virtually all HMOs offer resources such as recorded phone information on a huge range of health-related topics, along with hot lines staffed by nurses who can answer many of your other questions or help you determine if an office visit is indicated. Using these services means you can make the most of your visits by going only when it's appropriate, and by not wasting time asking questions for which you could easily get answers elsewhere.

Finally, if you are really unhappy, consider changing your health insurance to a fee for service plan, and be prepared to pay for extra time with your doctor, just as you would with an attorney or an accountant. It's a truism that we place a higher value on things we pay for than on those we get for free. This may, in fact, be a large part of the perceived problems people have with their health care providers (just something to think about).

Doctor and Patient, or Doctor versus Patient?

In a world of I-it relationships, many people seem to see doctors not as skilled professionals, but as obstacles standing between them and the treatment they have already decided they should have. That is, they think that curing what ails them is mainly a matter of getting access to the right substances or procedures, and that doctors do more to interfere with that process than they do to help it.

A perfect example of this is an incident that took place several years ago when I was working at an urgent care center, having recently sold my private practice. The management of this center believed that it should be partly urgent care and partly family practice, which fit with how I wanted to practice medicine. In reality, however, the repeat business was not much like a family practice, at least not the way I envisioned it. Rather, it consisted mainly of people who visited for their urgent care needs without establishing any kind of a relationship with the center or its staff. In this way, it was the same as people going to the local grocery store whenever they need groceries, but not establishing a relationship with the grocer for ongoing nutritional consultation or advice on how to use the store's products.

Under the circumstances, I would have been smart not to try to relate to these people as individuals with particular problems and needs, for that only added a layer of responsibility for them that was clearly beyond their concern or desire. Although some responded politely, most could not have cared less. They had come in with a problem, they wanted that problem solved, and they didn't particularly want my opinion. Given that my desire was to have actual (I-thou) relationships with my patients, I often found myself at loggerheads with them.

The ability to explain why sometimes the best treatment is no treatment is the mark of a physician who is both skilled and courageous.

One Sunday morning I entered an exam room and found a couple and their four-year-old daughter, who had just come from church. They were brightly scrubbed, nicely dressed, and keenly concerned about their child's illness, although obviously not so concerned that they couldn't wait till after church to come to the clinic. The little girl had a cough, stuffy nose, and mild sore throat, which were making her uncomfortable at night. She was not running a fever, was not wheezing, and did not appear to be suffering acute discomfort. After examining her, I determined that she had a cold. I prescribed the appropriate treatment: a decongestant for the stuffiness, something for the cough, and plenty of hot fluids (even chicken soup, which is wonderfully effective for colds). I offered the parents reassurance that the cold would go away in a few days to a week, and that she would do pretty well until that time.

Her father, however, was not satisfied with this response. "The child is sick," he said. "She needs an antibiotic."

I explained, I hope patiently, that an antibiotic was not indicated. Giving her an antibiotic would simply result in a pool of bacteria that would survive the onslaught and become stronger, thus being more resistant later when an antibiotic was really needed. I went on to explain that antibiotics, like armies, don't just kill the bad guys. They also kill the good guys. Where in the history of warfare has an army, however humane, been able to surgically root out the enemy and leave intact the lives and homes of innocent noncombatants?

Unfortunately, my little speech served only to annoy my patient's father. He reared up to his full 6′ plus height, looming over my slightly portly 5′4″ frame, and said menacingly that an antibiotic was what he came for, and an antibiotic was what he was going to get.

A man less foolish than myself would have said at this point, "Customer wants antibiotic, customer gets antibiotic," written a prescription, and sent him on his way. This reaction would have made everybody happy, including the manufacturer that makes the antibiotic; the organization that stocks it; the management that makes a profit off of it; the clinic that loves happy customers and wants repeat business; the nurses who like to see smiling faces when patients walk out the door; the patients who like to get what they want; and even the doctor who is respected for doing a bad job and is protected from an accumulation of complaints that would cause him to not have a job at all.

However, I did not take the politically correct (one might say "prudent") route. I knew I had given the most appropriate advice, which is finally being recognized as such in numerous articles in such prestigious journals as *JAMA* and the *New England Journal of Medicine,* and duly reported in local newspapers. So I stood by my principles and refused to prescribe the antibiotic, thereby incurring the wrath and discomfort of everybody, not the least myself, as the fallout reverberated throughout the system.

The best practitioner is one who is well versed in her own system of healing but also recognizes the existence of other models that can offer benefits to her patients.

This episode was a career-defining one for me as it underscored what I believe is the most important thing that a physician can do for a patient. When I ask myself the questions, "What would I want in a professional? What would I want in a physician?" several things come to mind, such as knowledge, skill, wisdom, kindness, and compassion. But the most important of these and the one that stands far and above any other qualities—is integrity. Compromising in order to comfort or pacify a patient, while knowing that the compromise would sooner or later prove detrimental to that patient, would ultimately make me a poorer doctor, as I would only make more compromises as time went on.

Society has empowered physicians with the rights and privileges of tending to the illnesses of its people. This is such a significant responsibility that for many years doctors were protected from the marketplace, even while we were being enriched by it, a situation I believe we heartily abused. Many of the upheavals that are occurring within conventional medicine, as well as the growth of alternative medicine, are a response to that abuse. Instead of trying to keep up with their craft and increasing their knowledge with information such as I am providing in this book, too many physicians have taken the expedient route of giving in to the desires of their clients. As a result, many have lost their integrity without even realizing that they have done so.

If a physician doesn't ask the questions, "How will this test help me make an accurate diagnosis?" or "What benefit will this medicine have for improving the patient's immediate condition and long-term health?" and then ask what treatment will provide the most short- and long-term benefit, then he risks not dealing with integrity. This is because every test has its risks—not to mention its costs—and all treatments have side effects, some of which are very, very damaging. Using tests without caution can be disastrous. A physician must be willing to do nothing at all, and to recommend that nothing be done, even in the face of some very uncomfortable symptoms. The ability to explain why sometimes the best treatment is no treatment is the mark of a physician who is both skilled and courageous.

What to Look For in a Healer

Although I have been discussing doctors and patients, what
I've been saying applies to any healer-patient relationship.
Medical doctors are the most common healers in this society,
but there are numerous others who practice outside the realm
of conventional medicine—the so-called alternative healers. I
have some difficulty with this term, especially with regard to
well-trained practitioners who are considered alternative only
because of their geographic presence in the United States. In
Germany, naturopaths are not alternative. Nor are those who
practice Ayurvedic medicine in India, or Chinese medicine in
China. We are the alternative practitioners in those countries.

Primary and Secondary Healers

What training, then, should you look for in a healer? I think of
this in terms of primary and secondary roles. In western conventional medicine, the person in the primary role is usually a
medical doctor. This is someone who is fully trained in all aspects of the body, health, and disease according to the western
medical model and the scientific method, and who uses various tools to manipulate the body. Such a practitioner knows
that all pharmacological substances, whether they are manufactured drugs, herbs, or supplements, have a physiological effect on the body that will show itself in physical, emotional,
and/or mental changes.

By contrast, an Ayurvedic practitioner starts from the
point of spirit, and uses spiritual, meditative, behavioral, and
herbal processes to achieve health. Chinese doctors work
with what they call the five element theory and use needles

(acupuncture), massage, and herbs to affect both the physical and etheric aspects of the body. All of these three types of practitioner are fully trained in their own systems of medical knowledge and know how to diagnose conditions and determine appropriate treatment within their respective realms. I call such people primary healers.

Both you and your healer should carefully consider your particular condition, needs, and health goals, along with the available information on SAMe, before deciding how to proceed. In any case, SAMe should be only one part of an overall approach that involves self-help strategies and various other therapies as appropriate.

The secondary healers are those who know aspects of those systems. The physical therapist is one such secondary healer. He understands an aspect of the general system in detail and possesses an overview of the entire system, though less completely than the medical doctor. Other examples of secondary healers include massage therapists, nurses, and nutritionists. All of these practitioners perform specific secondary functions that support the primary healing role.

Some people contend that naturopathy and homeopathy are primary healing systems. I can see the argument for that, although neither is as well grounded as the first three types of healers I mentioned. Some may even put chiropractic within the primary domain, and I know some chiropractors who believe that adjustments are all that are necessary even for such organic problems as heart disease. I don't believe, however, that most chiropractors hold this position.

Another type of practice that some perceive as primary is herbology. However, in my experience herbologists do not have complete knowledge of body systems so much as a utilitarian understanding of how specific herbs work for one condition or another. Personally, I place great value on their services, in the same way that I value pharmacologists and pharmacists as having a wide knowledge of medications that may affect my patients in positive (or negative) ways.

I firmly believe the best approach is to choose a primary healer who is *formally* trained in a major healing system. Probably because I come from the conventional western medical tradition, that is the first group I think of, but any alternative practitioner with full training would be appropriate. Once you have established this primary relationship, you can draw in secondary caregivers with the support and knowledge of the primary caregiver. This is not difficult if you are working with professionals who are all within the same system. For instance, if you are working with a doctor and also require the services of a physical therapist and a nutritionist, or even another primary physician such as a surgeon, you are not likely to meet much resistance about the players you choose for your team. The difficulty arises when you mix systems. If, for instance, you want a primary care physician, but you also want to work with an herbologist and another primary caregiver like an acupuncturist, then you need a primary care physician who is both open-minded and at least passingly familiar with the other systems, so that his own approach does not conflict with them.

The best practitioner is one who is well versed in her own system of healing but also recognizes the existence of other models that can offer benefits to her patients. This requires taking the time and effort to learn enough about the other systems to be able to work effectively alongside them, along with a willingness to recognize one's own limitations. As a family practitioner, I would not perform open heart surgery on a patient. I would leave that to someone with the training and experience to do so. In the same way, although I might support the use of acupuncture, I would not attempt to place the needles myself. Instead, I would send my patient to someone trained in those techniques.

Questions to Ask About the Healer

1. Is he trained at an accredited and recognized institution in his field?

2. Is he a primary healer, as defined above?

3. Does he recognize different fields and philosophies of healing other than his own?

4. How does he relate to those other fields and philosophies?

5. Does he interact with you?

6. Is he respectful of your perspective (this does not preclude challenging it in order to refine and strengthen it)?

Questions to Ask Yourself

1. What knowledge do you have to evaluate the healer's field of practice (the more you know, the more objective your evaluation will be)?

2. What do you want from your healer—total care and management, or consultation and advice?

3. What are your beliefs about healing, and how will they enhance or interfere with those of the healer?

4. Do you trust this person?

Discussing SAMe with Your Doctor

All of this being said, what if you have discovered a new substance, such as SAMe, and want to try it with the knowledge and support of your primary healer? Certainly it is appropriate to bring the subject up and provide as much information on it as you possibly can. Because SAMe is such a new substance (at least in the United States), the information on it, although good, is not splattered all over the medical literature. For that matter, there has not been much publicity about the detrimental effects of anti-inflammatories and the search for chondroprotective agents in general. By alerting your doctor to this information, you are doing him a great service. Keeping up with the changes in conventional medicine, much less with the wealth of alternative options, is a gargantuan task. Any physician with the qualities I've discussed here should appreciate help in that direction. In fact, your introduction is likely to spark a broader inquiry, as the doctor seeks out other information on the topic. This is one of the joys of an I-thou relationship. The learning goes in both directions.

If, on the other hand, a physician or other caregiver simply dismisses the information without reviewing it, you would have a good reason to look for a different practitioner. As I said before, there is so much knowledge available that anyone who claims to be a repository of all of it is clearly fooling herself and only demonstrating her own arrogance.

Both you and your healer should carefully consider your particular condition, needs, and health goals, along with the available information on SAMe, before deciding how to proceed. In any case, SAMe should be only one part of an overall approach that involves self-help strategies and various other therapies as appropriate. These include exercise and weight control for osteoarthritis; psychotherapy and antidepressants for depression; exercise and stress reduction for fibromyalgia; and treatment for alcohol abuse in the case of alcoholic liver cirrhosis.

CHAPTER 14

THE PHARMACOLOGY OF SAMe

How can one substance be effective in treating conditions as different from one another as osteoarthritis, depression, and liver disease? The answer lies in SAMe's unique chemical makeup. In essence, SAMe serves as a sort of molecular transport vehicle, carrying chemical components that it passes on to other molecules in order to facilitate various chemical reactions and produce a wide range of substances critical to body functions.

For those who are interested, this chapter provides a brief, high-level overview of SAMe's chemistry. It also investigates how different forms of SAMe are absorbed into and used by the body.*

---

* All the information in this chapter was derived from one source—an excellent article, titled "Pharmacologic Aspects of S-Adenosylmethionine," featured in the November 20, 1987, issue of the *American Journal of Medicine.*

The Chemistry of SAMe

As we have learned, our bodies manufacture S-adenosyl-methionine (SAMe) by combining the amino acid methionine with the "energy molecule," adenosine tri-phosphate (ATP), through the intervention of the enzyme S-adenomethionine synthetase (SAMe synthetase). This process creates a substance that is extremely reactive in the body, the primary feature of which is its ability to transfer one of its chemical components, called a methyl group, to other molecules in order to create new molecules. A methyl group is a hydrocarbon radical—a group of atoms that acts as a single atom in chemical reactions. Methyl radicals consist of one carbon atom and three hydrogen atoms, and thus have the formula CH_3. The process of transferring a methyl group from SAMe to another molecule is called methylation. In mammals, methylation occurs in some 40 different body processes.

By donating its methyl group, each SAMe molecule is converted to another substance called S-adenosyl-homocysteine or SAH. The SAH molecules, in turn, donate sulfur (the "S" portion) to other molecules in a process called transulfuration. Like methyl groups, sulfur is critical for numerous body processes, and SAH is one of the body's major sulfur donors. During transulfuration, the SAH also loses the adenosine group it inherited from the ATP, leaving straight homocysteine. (You may have heard about homocysteine in reference to its role in vascularization and heart disease. Although homocysteine seems to show promise for treating heart problems, that promise does not seem to apply to SAMe itself.)

Because ATP is universally present in the body, some researchers have speculated that taking methionine might enable increased production of SAMe and provide the same benefits as taking SAMe itself. Unfortunately, this has not been shown to be the case. This is too bad, since methionine is an abundant amino acid that can be found in health food stores at low cost. As I pointed out in Chapter 2, however, just because something is natural and available does not mean it is safe. In too large a dose, methionine can actually become toxic, leading to disorientation, vomiting, liver damage, and shock. The apparent reason for this is that the body limits the rate at which it combines methionine and ATP, causing toxic by-products of the reaction to build up to dangerous levels.

How SAMe Gets Absorbed into the Body

In order to be available for these complex chemical reactions, SAMe must first get into the bloodstream. Some substances, such as insulin, cannot be taken orally, because they are metabolized so quickly in the digestive tract that they never get a chance to be absorbed into the bloodstream. At the opposite end of this spectrum is glucose, which is absorbed into the bloodstream with incredible ease. Since glucose is the primary nutrient that the body needs to maintain itself, the intestine is specifically constructed to be able to break down whatever food substances come into it, in order to isolate the glucose and bring it into the general blood flow.

Fortunately, both the parenteral (or injectable) and oral versions of SAMe are readily accepted into the body. That is, enough SAMe gets through the digestive process to actually be absorbed into the bloodstream and become available for use. Oral administration does require higher doses because of the interference of the intestine.

Where Does It Go?

The amount of a substance that is absorbed into the blood-stream, as well as the length of time it remains there, is based on three factors:

- The substance's ability to maintain its structure before getting to the bloodstream

- The rate at which it is either metabolized by the liver or excreted by the kidneys

- The dosage—the higher the dose, the longer the substance is likely to remain in the bloodstream, or the stronger the "staying power"

A substance's "staying power" is measured by a unit called a half-life. The half-life is the amount of time it takes for a substance to reach half of its original concentration in the blood. For example, if the initial concentration of substance X is 50 micrograms per milliliter of blood, and five hours later the concentration is 25 micrograms per milliliter, the half-life of substance X is five hours.

Half-lives can be measured quite accurately with intravenous injections, because the initial concentration is also the peak concentration. Half-life measurements are not so accurate with medications that are given orally. It takes longer for the concentration to reach peak levels due to slower absorption, and even as the level is dropping from the original dose of the medication, more may be coming into the bloodstream. The half-life of SAMe, when administered intravenously, has been measured at approximately 81 minutes for a 100 mg dose, and 101 minutes for a 500 mg dose.[1]

Once in the blood, a substance can leave two ways. It can be metabolized (changed into a different substance) by the liver or it can be excreted by the kidneys. Consequently, one way to determine how well a substance is utilized in the body is to see whether and how much of it is secreted in the urine. The path of a substance through the blood can be measured by adding a chemical group or radioactive tag to the substance so that it can be easily detected in the urine. Experiments done by adding radioactive tags to SAMe showed that most of SAMe is used up in the body rather than being excreted. This, along with SAMe's short half-life in the blood, suggests that it is actually going directly to the areas in the body where it is most needed.

In essence, SAMe serves as a sort of molecular transport vehicle, carrying chemical components that it passes on to other molecules in order to facilitate various chemical reactions and produce a wide range of substances critical to body functions.

Kidney function itself is measured using an intravenous administration of a substance called inulin. Because inulin is not well metabolized in the body and is a small molecule, a person with healthy kidneys will excrete it fairly rapidly. Therefore, if the inulin does not show up in the expected amounts during a given period of time, the kidneys are not functioning properly.

Experimental Studies

Following is a sampling of the experimental data available on SAMe, including studies measuring absorption, effects on pain and swelling, and toxicity.

Absorption Rates

Various experiments have been done to measure how much SAMe is absorbed into the blood and how rapidly it is metabolized. As you would expect, administering SAMe intravenously causes its levels in the blood to rise very quickly. With oral administration, the levels rise much more slowly but are sustained over a longer period of time.

When taken orally, SAMe has a hard time getting past the stomach, but is more readily absorbed through the intestine. Researchers determined this by measuring the amount of SAMe in the portal system of the blood (the system that feeds into the liver) when SAMe was administered to rats two different ways, either orally or intraduodenally (bypassing the stomach). The difference was substantial. An oral dose of 32 mg per kilogram of body weight of SAMe resulted in a concentration of about four micrograms per milliliter of blood. The same dose given intraduodenally resulted in a concentration of 24 to 25 micrograms per milliliter—a six-fold increase.[1]

Fortunately, both the parenteral (or injectable) and oral versions of SAMe are readily accepted into the body. That is, enough SAMe gets through the digestive process to actually be absorbed into the bloodstream and become available for use.

Obviously administering SAMe intraduodenally is not a practical option for humans. However, the same effects can be accomplished by using an enteric-coated capsule, which protects the SAMe until it gets past the stomach. Researchers also found a difference in absorption when the enteric capsules were taken on an empty stomach versus a full stomach. In one experiment, dogs were given 100 mg enteric-coated capsules of SAMe. One group was given the capsules after an overnight fast, and the other group was given the capsules 30 minutes after eating, when the stomach is undergoing peak activity to digest the meal. The fasting group absorbed the SAMe faster and in greater quantities, with the highest plasma levels occurring between 40 minutes and two hours after ingestion. SAMe levels in the post-eating group rose more slowly and never reached the levels achieved by taking it on an empty stomach. This was balanced, however, by the SAMe being absorbed slowly, so that its levels continued to rise even six hours after administration. By contrast, in the fasting group, levels started to drop after two hours, and by six hours a very small amount of SAMe remained.[1]

Interestingly, men and women appear to absorb SAMe at different rates.

Interestingly, men and women appear to absorb SAMe at different rates. In an experiment in which men and women took 200 mg capsules of SAMe after an overnight fast, the women showed peak levels earlier than and higher than the men. The levels peaked at about three hours and lasted as long as six hours, with the peak levels being twice as high, on average, in women as in men.[1]

All of this demonstrates that SAMe is absorbed fairly well once it gets past the stomach, or when it is administered intravenously, and that it is well utilized in the body, but has a relatively short half-life. This means that people should not have to take more than two doses per day, which fits with the evidence from clinical studies.

Effect on Swelling and Pain

One experiment attempted to demonstrate SAMe's efficacy inside body tissues by measuring its anti-inflammatory activity in rats. The experimenters first gave the rats a substance called carrageenin to induce edema (swelling), which is a by-product of the inflammatory response. They then gave the rats either an intraduodenal dose of SAMe or an empty gelatin capsule, and measured the volume of edema several times over the next few hours. After two hours, the SAMe group showed 43.5 percent greater inhibition of edema than the control group. At three hours, the difference was 34.5 percent; at four hours, 32 percent; and at five hours, 29 percent. This suggests that the rats that were treated with SAMe had at least a one-third improvement in their edema level over the controls. The same experiment was repeated comparing SAMe with indomethacin. In this experiment, the indomethacin-treated group showed more improvement than the SAMe group, with both groups improving more than the control group.[1]

Three experiments tested SAMe's analgesic activity. Experimenters gave rats a pain-causing substance, either phenyl quinone or acetic acid, and observed how much of the substance was needed for the rats to show a pain response. They then administered SAMe or another test substance to a group of rats and measured how much of the pain-causing substance was needed to elicit the pain response in those rats. This showed them how well the test substance was able to inhibit pain.[1]

In one experiment, rats that received 200 mg of SAMe per kilogram of body weight showed a 71 percent greater inhibition of pain against phenyl quinone, as compared to the controls, and a 53 percent greater inhibition against acetic acid. A similar experiment tested SAMe against acetaminophen. Rats that received 50 mg of SAMe per kilogram of body weight showed a 60 percent improvement in pain, compared to a 15 percent improvement with acetaminophen. A third experiment, which used heat to elicit the pain response, compared 100 mg of SAMe per kilogram of body weight to 5 mg of morphine per kilogram. Just after administration, both the SAMe and morphine-treated groups reacted to the heat stimulus at about the same time—about five seconds. Thirty minutes after treatment, the SAMe group responded to the heat in 10.2 seconds, compared to the morphine group response of 19.8 seconds, and the control group response of 6.6 seconds. So, while it is not as effective a pain-killer as morphine, SAMe appears to hold its own against acetaminophen and is demonstrably better than nothing.[1]

Toxicity

As I discussed in the chapters on osteoarthritis, aspirin and the anti-inflammatories have some potentially nasty side effects, including gastrointestinal (GI) irritation, interference with blood clotting mechanisms, and inhibition of prostaglandin, a hormone involved in the body's inflammatory response.

The experimental evidence shows no such toxicity for SAMe. In one study using rats, a 1,200 mg per kilogram instillation of SAMe for 30 days had no effect on the integrity of the gastric mucosa (the lining of the digestive tract). In other words, SAMe does not adversely affect the protective mechanisms of the cells in GI tissues. Other experiments showed that SAMe does not influence platelet aggregation (clotting), which suggests that it presents no dangers for patients on Coumadin or other blood-thinners. Compared to indomethacin, SAMe can inhibit some prostaglandin activity, but only with a dose 1,500 times that of the indomethacin. In stark contrast to anti-inflammatories, SAMe does not interfere with the protective mechanisms in the cartilage; instead, because of its transulfuration into the proteoglycan, it seems to actually help it.[1]

. . . SAMe is absorbed fairly well once it gets past the stomach or when it is administered intravenously, and . . . is well utilized in the body, but has a relatively short half-life. This means that people should not have to take more than two doses per day . . .

In summary, the experimental data show that SAMe is well absorbed through the intramuscular and intravenous routes, and is reasonably well absorbed through the oral route, as long as an enteric-coated capsule is used. It maintains a sufficiently good half-life for therapeutic effect, and it shows essentially no toxicity.

Is There Such a Thing
As a Normal Level of SAMe?

I've mentioned a number of studies that have looked at measurements of SAMe in the body, particularly those that found correlations between low levels of SAMe and certain conditions. This may have caused you to wonder if there are tests for SAMe, and if so, whether you should get tested. After all, we can measure a person's level of thyroid stimulating hormone (TSH) to detect an underfunctioning thyroid gland, leading to treatment with levothyroxine (Synthroid), a synthetic form of thyroid hormone. But this analogy is a false one. Presumably, we could develop a clinical test to measure SAMe levels, but such measurements would have zero benefit. I'll say it as clearly as I can: There is no direct relationship between low levels of SAMe and the therapeutic benefits of taking it. In fact, as we have seen, in at least one condition where low levels of SAMe were found—that is, in the central nervous system of persons with Parkinson's disease—the use of SAMe offered equivocal benefits.

Unlike hormones, which have a direct and observable effect on the body, the connection between chemical reactions that happen at a molecular level and what happens at the clinical level—that is, what we can detect in the body through tests or observation—is questionable in almost every way. Despite this fact, some practitioners attempt to manipulate levels of various substances in the mistaken belief that "normal levels" somehow equate to being healthy.

There is no direct relationship between low levels of SAMe and the therapeutic benefits of taking it.

An extreme example of this was a chiropractor who would draw blood samples in order to check his patients' levels of sodium, potassium, chloride, glucose, blood urea nitrogen (BUN), carbon dioxide, and creatinine. He would then proceed to give the patient various substances in an attempt to manipulate the numbers to match the exact mean. For example, if a person's sodium was 140, and the "normal" range was 140 to 150, he would attempt to get the sodium level to 145. Anyone who knows much about physiology recognizes the foolishness of this process. The body's self-regulation system is extremely efficient, and such supplementation changes levels for a very short period of time, if at all.

The more pertinent question is, what does changing a person's sodium level do to help their general health and well-being? The answer is, nothing. I remember making jokes (admittedly somewhat macabre ones) about patients in the intensive care unit whose electrolytes were way out of whack. We worked very hard to put them into order, even when we knew that a patient's demise was both inevitable and imminent. The joke went, "The numbers were perfect when the patient died."

Unlike synthetic hormones such as Synthroid or estrogen substitutes, the purpose of taking SAMe is not to raise the ambient level of SAMe in the body. Instead, the purpose is to load the system with higher levels of raw material, in order to enhance a process that is already working. Taking SAMe is similar to taking a substance like tryptophan. Under normal circumstances, tryptophan acts as a precursor to certain neurotransmitters, particularly serotonin. When you load the system with tryptophan, this "pushes the reaction to the right"; that is, the body tends to equalize out the tryptophan by manufacturing more serotonin. Similarly, when you load the system with SAMe, you increase the supply of methyl donors. The body then uses the extra supply where it is most needed, as part of its innate self-regulating process.

FUTURE
DIRECTIONS

We've seen in this book that S-adenosylmethionine—SAMe—is a legitimate contender for playing a part in the new age of therapeutics. To that end, it has several factors working in its favor:

- It is made in the body. Consequently, taking SAMe does not lead to toxicity as many exogenous substances can, because the body has so many mechanisms that can regulate its use.

- Its mechanisms in the body are widespread. We can see SAMe's involvement—through methylation and sulfuration—in just about every aspect of the body's metabolism.

- Some of its specific functions provide direct benefits in specific disease states—certainly for osteoarthritis and cirrhosis of the liver, probably for depression, and possibly Alzheimer's disease. The effectiveness of SAMe is probably

primarily because SAMe increases cell membrane permeability, but also because it has some reparative effect, especially in osteoarthritis.

• It is relatively non-toxic. It is true that whenever you load
any kind of a system with too much of any kind of a substance, the chances of toxicity are greatly increased. However, the evidence demonstrates that SAMe is not very toxic
even when taken in high doses. And it is clearly far less toxic
than any of the drugs that would be used in its place.

. . . the evidence demonstrates that SAMe is not very toxic even when taken in high doses.

Where SAMe still falls short, unfortunately, is in its high
cost. Although various attempts have been made to reduce the
cost of manufacturing SAMe, the limited demand for it has not
created an impetus to pursue such attempts with any degree of
rigor. I believe, however, that this may change once people
start to recognize SAMe's myriad benefits.[1-3]

Directions for Future Research

Although it would be quite appropriate to search for other
possible benefits of SAMe, directing research to the avenues

that show the most promise at this point will give us more "bang for the buck." Consequently, we should be paying a lot more attention to what SAMe can do for osteoarthritis and cirrhosis of the liver, particularly over the long term. To a lesser extent, it would be worthwhile to pursue research on depression and Alzheimer's disease, as well.

. . . SAMe should and will play a significant role, not only in the treatment of specific diseases, but as a spearhead for a whole new class of bioactive substances that will prove to be of greater benefit and less toxicity than the drugs we are working with today.

Osteoarthritis

Research on SAMe and OA should be geared toward determining whether SAMe is actually chondroprotective, and if so to what extent. This would require long-term clinical studies lasting at least six months to a year. The studies should include thorough examinations and measurements of the arthritic joints at both the beginning and the end of the study, in order to determine the amount of repair, if any. The evidence, both anecdotal and experimental, certainly warrants individual use of SAMe for osteoarthritis even now. But a process of long-term research could open a door for a much better class of drug than currently exists for people suffering from osteoarthritis.

Cirrhosis of the Liver

As with OA, we don't really know much about SAMe's reparative effects on the liver and whether it could actually overcome a lot of the damage done by alcohol, drugs, and other causes. Taking liver biopsies before and after a long-term trial of SAMe—one lasting six months to a year or more—may help to answer those questions.

Alzheimer's Disease

As I pointed out in Chapter 12, to date there have not been any good clinical studies to determine whether SAMe has any effect whatsoever on Alzheimer's disease. I don't believe, however, that it would be possible to see any significant effects in a trial shorter than six months.

Depression

Depression is a somewhat different story. The evidence clearly shows that SAMe can relieve or lessen depressive symptoms in the short term. However, a lot of substances can be beneficial for depression, and SAMe might not be the highest on the list. For mild depression, St. John's wort is probably at least as effective, and certainly much cheaper. For long-term treatment of severe depression, the tricyclics are probably still the best option, followed closely by the SSRIs. However, as we've seen, SAMe is much less toxic and more readily tolerated than either of these. If it were to become available at a reasonable cost, SAMe could become the treatment of choice for long-term treatment of depression. However, since there have not been any long-term studies, we don't know if SAMe's benefits are self-limiting and whether higher doses over a period of time would be less effective. This again underscores the need for long-term clinical trials.

New Directions

It's important to remember that all of these diseases, especially depression, involve multiple factors. In treating any disease, we must deal with all of its aspects, rather than relying solely on drugs or supplements. There is no doubt in my mind, however, that SAMe should and will play a significant role, not only in the treatment of specific diseases, but as a spearhead for a whole new class of bio-active substances that will prove to be of greater benefit and less toxicity than the drugs we are working with today.

NOTES

Chapter 1

1. Lazarou, J. and Pomeranz, B., "Incidence of Adverse Drug Reactions in Hospitalized Patients: A Meta-Analysis of Prospective Studies" *Journal of American Medicine* (15 April 1998): 279 (15): 1200-5.
2. Cozens, D.D., et al., "Reproductive Toxicity Studies of Ademetionine" *Arzneitmittel-Forschung* (November 1988): 38 (11): 1625-9.
3. Pezzoli, C., Galli-Kienle, M., and Stramentinoli, G., "Lack of Mutagenic Activity of Ademetionine in Vitro and in Vivo" *Arzneitmittel-Forschung* (July 1987): 37 (7): 826-9.
4. Charlton, C.G., and Crowell, B., Jr., "Parkinson's Disease-Like Effects of S-Adenosyl-L-Methionine: Effects of L-Dopa" *Pharmacology, Biochemistry & Behavior* (October 1992): 43 (2): 423-31.
5. Rakasz, E., Sugar, J., and Csuka, O., "Modulation of Cytosine Arabinoside-Induced Proliferation Inhibition by Exogenous Adenosylmethionine" *Cancer Chemotherapy & Pharmacology* (1991): 28 (6): 484-6.

Chapter 3

1. Garber, A.M., Browner, W.S., and Hulley, S.B., "Cholesterol Screening in Asymptomatic Adults, Revisited. Part 2" *Annals of Internal Medicine* (March 1996): 124 (5): 518-31.
2. Criqui, M.H., "Cholesterol, Primary and Secondary Prevention, and All-Cause Mortality" *Annals of Internal Medicine* (15 December 1991): 115 (12): 973-6.
3. Jenkins, C.D., "Psychologic and Social Precursors of Coronary Disease" *New England Journal of Medicine* (4 February 1971): 284 (5): 244-55.

Chapter 6

1. Bassleer, C., Gysen, P., Bassleer, R., and Franchimont, P., "Proteoglycans Synthesized by Human Chondrocytes Cultivated in Clusters" *American Journal of Medicine* (20 November 1987): 83 (5a): 25-28.
2. Floman, Y., Eyre, D.R., and Glimcher, M.J., "Induction of Osteoarthritis in the Rabbit Knee Joint: Biochemical Studies on the Articular Cartilage" *Clinical Orthopaedics & Related Research* (March–April 1980): (147): 278-86.
3. Cox, M.J., McDevitt, C.A., Arnoczky, S.P., and Warren, R.F., "Changes in the Chondroitin Sulfate-Rich Region of Articular Cartilage Proteoglycans in Experimental Osteoarthritis" *Biochimica et Biophysica Acta* (18 June 1985): 840 (2): 228-34.
4. Floman, Y., 278-86.
5. Thompson, R.C., Jr., and Oegema, T.R., Jr., "Metabolic Activity of Articular Cartilage in Osteoarthritis, an In-Vitro Study" *Journal of Bone & Joint Surgery—American Volume* (April 1979): 61 (3): 407-16.
6. Vignon, E., Chapuy, M.C., Arlot, M., Richard, M., Louisot, P., and Vignon, G., "Study of the Concentration of Glycosaminoglycans in Cartilage from Normal and Osteoarthritic Femoral Head" *Pathologie Biologie* (April 1975): 23 (4): 283-9.

Notes

7. Sweet, M.B., Thonar, E.J., Immelman, A.R., and Solomon, L., "Biochemical Changes in Progressive Osteoarthrosis" *Annals of Rheumatic Diseases* (October 1977): 36 (5): 387-98.

8. Shield, M.J., "Anti-Inflammatory Drugs and Their Effects on Cartilage Synthesis and Renal Function" *European Journal of Rheumatology & Inflammation* (1993): 13 (1): 7-16.

9. Brandt, K., "Should Osteoarthritis Be Treated with Nonsteroidal Anti-Inflammatory Drugs?" *Rheumatic Diseases Clinics of North America* (August 1992): 19 (3): 697-712.

10. Brandt, K., "Effects of Nonsteroidal Anti-Inflammatory Drugs on Chondrocyte Metabolism in Vitro and in Vivo" *American Journal of Medicine* (20 November 1987): 83 (5a): 29-35.

11. Adams, M.E., "Cartilage Research and Treatment of Osteoarthritis" *Current Opinion on Rheumatology* (August 1992): 4 (4): 552-9.

12. Lewandowski, B., Bernacka, K., Cylwik, B., Duda, D., Klimiuk, P.A., "Piroxicam and Poststeroidal Damage of Articular Cartilage" (1995): *Roczniki Akademii Medycznej W Bialymstoku* 40 (2): 396-408.

13. Rainsford, K.D., "Mechanisms of NSAIDs on Joint Destruction in Osteoarthritis" *Agents and Actions—Supplements* (1993): 44: 39-43.

14. Dingle, J.T., "Cartilage Maintenance in Osteoarthritis: Interaction of Cytokines, NSAID and Prostaglandins in Articular Cartilage Damage and Repair" *Journal of Rheumatology—Supplement* (March 1991): 28: 30-7.

15. Bassleer, C.T., Henrotin, Y.E., Regnister, J.L., and Franchimont, P.P., "Effects of Tiaprofenic Acid and Acetylsalicylic Acid on Human Articular Chondrocytes in 3-Dimensional Culture" *Journal of Rheumatology* (September 1992): 19 (9): 1433-8.

16. Henrotin, Y., Bassleer, C., and Franchimont, P., "In Vitro Effects of Etrodolac and Acetylsalicylic Acid on Human Chondrocyte Metabolism" *Agents & Actions* (July 1992): 36 (3-4): 317-23.

17. Malemud, C. Shuckett, J.R., and Goldberg, V.M., "Changes in Proteoglycans of Human Osteoarthritic Cartilage Maintained in Explant Culture: Implications for Understanding Repair in Osteoarthritis" *Scandinavian Journal of Rheumatology—Supplement* (1988): 77: 7-12.

18. Worrall, J.G., Wilkinson, L.S., Bayliss, M.T., and Edwards, J.C., "Zonal Distribution of Chondroitin-4-Sulphate/Dermatan Sulphate and Chondroitin-6-Sulphate in Normal and Diseased Human Synovium" *Annals of the Rheumatic Diseases* (January 1994): 53 (1): 35-8.

19. Ratcliffe, A., Billingham, M.E., Saed-Nejad, F., Muir, H., and Hardingham, T.E., "Increased Release of Matrix Components from Articular Cartilage in Experimental Canine Osteoarthritis" *Journal of Orthopaedic Research* (May 1992): 10 (3): 350-8.

20. Manicourt, D.H., Druetz-Van Egeren, A., Haazen, L., and Nagant De Deuxchaisnes C., "Effects of Tenoxicam and Aspirin on the Metabolism of Proteoglycans and Hyaluronan in Normal and Osteoarthritic Human Articular Cartilage" *British Journal of Pharmacology* (December 1994): 113 (4): 1113-20.

21. Fassbender, H., "Role of Chondrocyte in the Development of Osteoarthritis" *American Journal of Medicine* (20 November 1987): 83 (5a): 17-24.

22. Setnikar, I., "Antireactive Properties of 'Chondroprotective' Drugs" *International Journal of Tissue Reactions* (1992): 14 (5): 253-61.

23. Ito, A., and Mori, Y., "Effect of a Novel Anti-Inflammatory Drug" *Research Communications in Chemical Pathology and Pharmacology* (November 1990): 70 (2): 131-42.

Notes

24. A Whole Supplement Was Devoted to the Subject: *American Journal of Medicine—Supplement* (20 November 1987).

25. di Padova, C., "S-Adenosylmethionine in the Treatment of Osteoarthritis. Review of the Clinical Studies" *American Journal of Medicine* (20 November 1987): 83 (5a): 60-5.

26. Kalbhen, D.A., and Jansen, G., "Pharmacologic Studies on the Antidegenerative Effect of Ademetionine in Experimental Arthritis in Animals" *Arzneimittel-Forschung* (September 1990): 40 (9): 1017-21.

27. Barcelo, H.A., Weimeyer, J.C., Sagasta, C.L., Macias, M., and Barriera, J.C., "Experimental Osteoarthritis and Its Course When Treated with S-Adenosyl-L-Methionine" *Revista Clinica Espanola* (June 1990): 187 (2): 74-8.

28. Barcelo, H.A., Wiemeyer, J.C., Sagasta, C.L., Macias, M., and Barriera, J.C., "Effect of S-Adenosylmethionine on Experimental Osteoarthritis in Rabbits" *American Journal of Medicine* (20 November 1987): 83 (5a): 55-9.

29. Berger, R., and Nowak, H., "A New Medical Approach to the Treatment of Osteoarthritis. Report of an Open Phase IV Study with Ademetionine (Gumbaral)" *American Journal of Medicine* (20 November 1987): 83 (5a): 8408.

30. Konig, B., "A Long-Term (Two Years) Clinical Trial with S-Adenosylmethionine for the Treatment of Osteoarthritis" *American Journal of Medicine* (November 1987): 83 (5a): 89-94, 20.

31. Domljan, Z., Vrhovac, B., Durrigl, T., and Pucar, I., "A Double-Blind Trial of Ademetionine vs. Naproxen in Activated Gonarthrosis" *International Journal of Clinical Pharmacology, Therapy & Toxicology* (July 1989): 27 (7): 329-33.

32. Caruso, I. and Pietrogrande, V., "Italian Double-Blind Multicenter Study Comparing S-Adenosylmethionine Naproxen, and Placebo in the Treatment of Degenerative Joint Disease" *American Journal of Medicine* (20 November 1987): 83 (5a): 66-71.

33. Muller-Fassbender, H., "Double-Blind Clinical Trial of S-Adenosylmethionine Versus Ibuprofen in the Treatment of Osteoarthritis" *American Journal of Medicine* (20 November 1987): 83 (5a): 81-3.

34. Glorioso, S., Todesco, S., Mazzi, A., Marcolongo, R., Giordano, M., Colombo, B., Chrie-Ligniere, B.G., Mattara, L., Leardini, G., Passeri, M., et al., "Double-Blind Multicentre Study of the Activity of S-Adenosylmethionine in Hip and Knee Osteoarthritis" *International Journal of Clinical Pharmacology Research* (1985): 5 (1): 39-49.

35. Vetter, G., "Double-Blind Comparative Clinical Trial with S-Adenosylmethionine and Indomethacin in the Treatment of Osteoarthritis" *American Journal of Medicine* (20 November 1987): 83 (5a): 78-80.

36. Polli, E., Cortellaro, M., Parrini, L., Tessari, L., and Ligniere, G.C., "Pharmacological and Clinical Aspects of S-Adenosylmethionine (SAMe) in Primary Degenerative Arthropathy (Osteoarthritis)" *Minerva Medica* (5 December 1975): 66 (83): 4443-59.

37. Maccagno, A., DiGiorgio, E.E., Caston, O.L., and Sagasta, C.L., "Double-Blind Controlled Clinical Trial of Oral S-Adenosylmethionine versus Piroxicam in Knee Osteoarthritis" *American Journal of Medicine* (20 November 1987): 83 (5a): 72-7.

38. Bradley, J.D., Flusser, D., Katz, B.P., Schumacher, H.R., Jr., Brandt, K.D., Chambers, M.A., and Zonay, L. J., "A Randomized, Double-Blind, Placebo-Controlled Trial of Intravenous Loading with S-Adenosylmethionine (SAM) Followed by Oral SAM Therapy in Patients with Knee Osteoarthritis" *Journal of Rheumatology* (1994): 21 (5): 905-11.

Notes

39. Montrone, F., Fumagalli, M., Sarzi Puttini, P., Boccassini, L., Santandrea, S., Volpato, R., Locati, M., and Caruso I., "Double-Blind Study of S-Adenosyl-Methionine versus Placebo in Hip and Knee Arthrosis" *Clinical Rheumatology* (December 1985): 4 (4): 484-5.

40. Murray, M. *Encyclopedia of Nutritional Supplements.* Sacramento, CA: Prima Publishing, (1996).

41. Thompson, R.C., Jr., 407-16.

42. Sweet, M.B., 387-98.

43. Malemud, C., 7-12.

44. Worrall, J.G., 35-8.

45. Ratcliffe, A., 350-8.

46. Vignon, E., 283-9.

47. Karube, S. and Shoji, H., "Compositional Changes of Glycosaminoglycans of the Human Menisci with Age and Degenerative Joint Disease" *Nippon Seikeigeka Gakkai Zasshi—Journal of Japanese Orthopedic Association* (January 1982): 56 (1): 51-7.

48. Lopes, V. A. "Double-Blind Clinical Evaluation of the Relative Efficacy of Ibuprofen and Glucosamine Sulphate in the Management of Osteoarthrosis of the Knee in Out-Patients" *Current Medical Research & Opinion* (1982): 8 (3): 145-9.

49. D'Ambrosio, E., Casa, B., Bompani, R., Scali, G., and Scali, M. "Glucosamine Sulphate: A Controlled Clinical Investigation in Arthrosis" *Pharmatherapeutica* (1981): 2 (8): 504-8.

50. Reichelt, A., Forster, K.K., Fischer, M., Rovati, L.C., and Setnikar, I., "Efficacy and Safety of Intramuscular Glucosamine Sulfate in Osteoarthritis of the Knee. A Randomised, Placebo-Controlled, Double-Blind Study" *Arzneimittel-Forschung* (January 1994): 44 (1): 75-80.

51. Theodosakis, J., Adderly, B., and Fox, B., *The Arthritis Cure.* New York: St. Martin's Press (1997).

Chapter 9

1. Bottiglieri, T., Godfrey, P., Flynn, T., Carney, M.W., Toone, B.K., and Reynolds, E.H., "Cerebrospinal Fluid S-Adenosylmethionine in Depression and Dementia: Effects of Treatment with Parenteral and Oral S-Adenosylmethionine" *Journal of Neurology, Neurosurgery & Psychiatry* (December 1990): 53 (12): 1096-8.

2. Baldessarini, R.J., "Neuropharmacology of S-Adenosyl-L-Methionine" *American Journal of Medicine* (20 November 1987): 83 (5a): 95-103.

3. Bottiglieri, T., Hyland, K., and Reynolds, E.H., "The Clinical Potential of Ademetionine (S-Adenosylmethionine) in Neurological Disorders" *Drugs* (August 1994): 48 (2): 137-52.

4. Sitaram, B.R., Sitaram, M., Traut, M., and Chapman, C.B., "Nyctohemeral Rhythm in the Levels of S-Adenosylmethionine in the Rat Pineal Gland and Its Relationship to Melatonin Biosynthesis" *Journal of Neurochemistry* (October 1995): 65 (4): 1887-94.

5. Taylor, K.M., and Randall, P.K., "Depletion of S-Adenosyl-L-Methionine in Mouse Brain by Antidepressive Drugs" *Journal of Pharmacological Experimental Therapeutics* (1975): 194: 303-10.

6. Hietala, O.A., Laitinen, S.I., Laitinen, P.H., Lapinjoki, S.P., and Pajunen, A.E., "The Inverse Changes of Mouse Brain Ornithine and S-Adenosylmethionine

Notes

Decarboxylase Activities by Chlorpromazine and Imipramine. Dependence of Ornithine Decarboxylase Induction on Beta-Adrenoreceptors" *Biochemical Pharmacology* (1983): 32: 1581-5.

7. Monaco, P., and Quattrocchi, F., "Study of the Antidepressive Effects of a Biological Transmethylating Agent (S-Adenosylmethionine or SAM)" *Rivista De Neurologia* (November-December 1979): 49 (6): 417-39.

8. Fava, M., Rosenbaum, J.F., MacLaughlin, R., Falk, W.E., Pollack, M.H., Cohen, L.S., Jones, L.L., and Pill, L., "Neuroendocrine Effects of S-Adenosyl-L-Methionine, A Novel Putative Antidepressant" *Journal of Psychiatric Research* (1990): 24 (2): 177-84.

9. Pinzello, A., and Andreoli, V., "Le Transmetilazioni SAM-Dipendenti Nelle Sindromi Depressive. Valutazione Dell-Effetto Terapeutico Dell S-Adenosilmethionina Con La Scala Di Hamilton" *Quad Ter Sper Suppl Bioch Biol Sper* (1972): X/2: 3-11.

10. Andreoli, V.M., Maffei, F., and Tonon, G.C., "S-Adenosyl-L-Methionine (SAMe) Blood Levels in Schizophrenia and Depression" *Monographien Aus Dem Gesamtgebiete Der Psychiatrie. Psychiatry Series* (1978): 18: 147-50.

11. Bressa, G.M., "S-Adenosyl-L-Methionine (SAMe) As Antidepressant: Meta-Analysis of Clinical Studies" *Acta Neurologica Scandinavica Supplement* (1994): 154: 7-14.

12. Jacobsen, S., Danneskiold-Samsoe, B., and Andersen, R.B., "Oral S-Adenosylmethionine in Primary Fibromyalgia. Double-Blind Clinical Evaluation" *Scandinavian Journal of Rheumatology* (1991): 20 (4): 294-302.

13. Bressa, G.M., 7-14.

14. Fava, M., Fiannelli, A., Rapisarda, V., Patralia, A., and Guaraldi, G.P., "Rapidity of Onset of the Antidepressant Effect of Parenteral S-Adenosyl-L-Methionine" *Psychiatry Research* (28 April 1995): 56 (3): 295-7.

15. Berlanga, C., Ortega-Soto, H.A., Ontiveros, M., and Senties H., "Efficacy of S-Adenosyl-L-Methionine in Speeding the Onset of Action of Imipramine" *Psychiatry Research* (December 1992): 44 (3): 257-62.

16. Lin, Y., "Acupuncture Treatment for Insomnia and Acupuncture Analgesia" *Psychiatry & Clinical Sciences* (May 1995): 49 (2): 119-20.

Chapter 10

1. Pisi, E., and Marchesini, G., "Mechanisms and Consequences of the Impaired Trans-Sulphuration Pathway in Liver Disease: Part II. Clinical Consequences and Potential for Pharmacological Intervention in Cirrhosis" *Drugs* (1990): 40 Suppl 3: 65-72.

2. Angelico, M., Gandin, C., Nistri, A., Baiocchi, L., and Capocaccia L., "Oral S-Adenosyl-L-Methionine (SAMe) Administration Enhances Bile Salt Conjugation with Taurine in Patients with Liver Cirrhosis" *Scandinavian Journal of Clinical & Laboratory Investigation* (October 1994): 54 (6): 459-64.

3. Pisi, E., 65-72.

4. Duce, A.M., Oritz, P., Cabrero, C., and Mato, J.M., "S-Adenosyl-L-Methionine Synthetase and Phospholipid Methyltransferase Are Inhibited in Human Cirrhosis" *Hepatology* (January–February 1988): 8 (1): 65-8.

5. Barak, A.J., Beckenhauer, H.C., Tuma, D.J., and Badakhsh, S., "Effects of Prolonged Ethanol Feeding on Methionine Metabolism in Rat Liver" *Biochemistry and Cell Biology* (March 1987): 65 (3): 230-3.

6. Miglio, F., Stefanini, G.F., Corazza, G.R., D'Ambro, A., and Gasbarrini, G., "Double-Blind Studies of the Therapeutic Action of S-Adenosylmethionine

Notes

(SAMe) in Oral Administration in Liver Cirrhosis and Other Chronic Hepatitidies" *Minerva Medica* (2 May 1995): 66 (33): 1595-9.

7. Labo, G., Miglio, F.D., D'Ambro, A., Bellobuono, A., Ideo, G., Dioguardi, N., Bernardi, M., Corazza, G.R., Gasbarrini, G., Avogaro, P., and Pasquino M., "Double-Blind Polycentric Study of the Action of S-Adenosylmethionine in Hepatic Cirrhosis" *Minerva Medica* (2 May 1975): 66 (33): 1590-4.

8. Cantoni, L., Maggi, G., Mononi, G., and Preti, G., "Relations Between Protidopoiesis and Biological Transmethylations: Action of S-Adenosylmethionine on Protein Crasis in Chronic Hepatopathies" *Minerva Medica* (2 May 1975): 66 (33): 1581-9.

9. Ideo, G., "S-Adenosylmethionine: Plasma Levels in Hepatic Cirrhosis and Preliminary Results of Its Clinical Use in Hepatology. Double-Blind Study" *Minerva Medica* (May 1975): 66 (33): 1571-80.

10. Colell, A., Garcia-Ruiz, C., Morales, A., Ballesta, A., Ookhtens, M., Rodes, J., Kaplowitz, N., and Fernandez-Checa, J.C., "Transport of Reduced Glutathione in Hepatic Mitochondria and Mitoplasts from Ethanol-Treated Rats: Effect of Membrane Physical Properties and S-Adenosyl-L-Methionine" *Hepatology* (September 1997): 26 (3): 699-708.

11. Kakimoto, H., Kawata, S., Imaim, Y., Inada, M., Matsuzawa, Y., and Tarui, S., "Changes in Lipid Composition of Erythrocyte Membranes with Administration of S-Adenosyl-L-Methionine in Chronic Liver Disease" *Gastroenterologia Japonica* (August 1992): 27 (4): 508-13.

12. Loguercio, C., Nardi, G., Argenzio, F., Aurilio, C., Petrone, E., Grella, A., Del Vecchio Blance, C., and Coltorti, M., "Effect of S-Adenosyl-L-Methionine Administration on Red Blood Cell Cysteine and Glutathione Levels in Alcoholic Patients With and Without Liver Disease" *Alcohol & Alcoholism* (September 1994): 29 (5): 597-604.

Chapter 11

1. Bennett, R.M., "Fibromyalgia: The Commonest Cause of Widespread Pain" *Comprehensive Therapy* (June 1995): 21 (6): 269-75.

2. Reveille, J.D., "Soft-Tissue Rheumatism: Diagnosis and Treatment" *American Journal of Medicine* (January 1997): 102 (1a): 23s-29s, 27.

3. Wallace, D.J., "The Fibromyalgia Syndrome" *Annals of Medicine* (February 1997): 29 (1): 9-21.

4. Wolfe, F., and Potter, J., "Fibromyalgia and Work Disability: Is Fibromyalgia a Disabling Disorder?" *Rheumatic Diseases Clinics of North America* (May 1996): 22 (2): 369-91.

5. Wallace, D.J., 9-21

6. Auvenshine, R.C., "Psychoneuroimmunology and Its Relationship to the Differential Diagnosis of Temporomandibular Disorders" *Dental Clinics of North America* (April 1997): 41 (2): 279-96.

7. Lowe, J.C., Cullum, M.E., Graf, L.H., Jr., and Yellin, J., "Mutations in the C-Erba Beta 1 Gene: Do They Underlie Euthyroid Fibromyalgia?" *Medical Hypotheses* (February 1997) 48 (2): 125-35.

8. Crofford, L.J., Engleberg, N.C., and Demitrack, M.A., "Neurohormonal Perturbations in Fibromyalgia" *Baillieres Clinical Rheumatology* (1996 May): 10 (2): 365-78.

9. Goldenberg, D.L., "Fibromyalgia, Chronic Fatigue Syndrome, and Myofascial Pain" *Current Opinion in Rheumatology* (March 1996): 8 (2): 113-23.

Notes

10. Wolfe, F., "Post-Traumatic Fibromyalgia: A Case Report Narrated by the Patient" *Arthritis Care & Research* (September 1994): 7 (3): 161-5.
11. Olin, R., "Fibromyalgia. A Neuro-Immuno-Endocrinologic Syndrome?" *Lakartidningen* (22 February 1995): 92 (8): 755-8, 761-3.
12. Modolfsky, H., "Sleep, Neuroimmune and Neuroendocrine Functions in Fibromyalgia and Chronic Fatigue Syndrome" *Advances in Neuroimmunology* (1995): 5 (1): 39-56.
13. Branco, J.C., "The Diagnosis and Treatment of Fibromyalgia" *Acta Medica Portuguesa* (April 1995): 8 (4): 233-8.
14. Clauw, D.J., "Fibromyalgia: More Than Just a Musculoskeletal Disease" *American Family Physician* (1 September 1995): 52 (3): 843-51, 853-4.
15. Hudson, J.I., and Pope, H.G., Jr., "The Relationship Between Fibromyalgia and Major Depressive Disorder" *Rheumatic Diseases Clinics of North America* (May 1996): 22 (2): 285-303.
16. Gruber, A.J., Hudson, J.L., and Pope, H.G., Jr., "The Management of Treatment-Resistant Depression in Disorders on the Interface of Psychiatry and Medicine. Fibromyalgia, Chronic Fatigue Syndrome, Migraine, Irritable Bowel Syndrome, Atypical Facial Pain, and Premenstrual Dysphoric Disorder" *Psychiatric Clinics of North America* (June 1996): 19 (2): 351-69.
17. Goodnick, P.J., and Sandoval, R., "Psychotropic Treatment of Chronic Fatigue Syndrome and Related Disorders" *Journal of Clinical Psychiatry* (January 1993): 54 (1): 13-20.
18. Bennett, R.M., "Multidisciplinary Group Programs to Treat Fibromyalgia Patients" *Rheumatic Diseases Clinics of North America* (May 1996): 22 (2): 351-67.
19. Buchwald, D., "Fibromyalgia and Chronic Fatigue Syndrome: Similarities and Differences" *Rheumatic Diseases Clinics of North America* (May 1996): 22 (2): 219-43.
20. Wilke, W.S., "Fibromyalgia: Recognizing and Addressing the Multiple Interrelated Factors" *Postgraduate Medicine* (July 1996): 100 (1): 153-6, 159, 163-6.
21. Rosen, N.B., "Physical Medicine and Rehabilitation Approaches to the Management of Myofascial Pain and Fibromyalgia Syndromes" *Baillieres Clinical Rheumatology* (November 1994): 8 (4): 881-916.
22. Jacobsen, S., Danneskiold-Samsoe, B., and Andersen, R.B., "Oral S-Adenosylmethionine in Primary Fibromyalgia-Double-Blind Clinical Evaluation" *Scandinavian Journal of Rheumatology* (1991): 20 (4): 294-302.
23. Volkmann, H., Norregaard, J., Jacobsen, S., Danneskiold-Samsoe, B., Knoke, G., and Nehrdich, D., "Double-Blind, Placebo-Controlled Cross-Over Study of Intravenous S-Adenosyl-L-Methionine in Patients with Fibromyalgia" *Scandinavian Journal of Rheumatology* (1997): 26 (3): 206-11.
24. Tavoni, A., Vitali, C., Bonbardieri, S., and Pasero, G., "Evaluation of S-Adenosylmethionine in Primary Fibromyalgia. A Double-Blind Crossover Study" *American Journal of Medicine* (20 November 1987): 83 (5a): 107-10.

Chapter 12

1. Charlton, C.G. and Crowell, B., Jr., "Striatal Dopamine Depletion, Tremors, and Hypokinesia Following the Intracranial Injection of S-Adenosylmethionine: A Possible Role of Hypermethylation in Parkinsonism" *Molecular & Chemical Neuropathology* (December 1995): 26 (3): 269-84.
2. Crowell, B.G., Jr., Benson, R., Shockley, D., and Charlton, C.G., "S-Adenosyl-L-Methionine Decreases Motor Activity in the Rat: Similarity to Parkinson's Disease-Like Symptoms" *Behavioral & Neural Biology* (May 1993): 59 (3): 186-93.

Notes

3. Geller, A.M., Kotb, M.Y., Jernigan, H.M., Jr., and Kredich, N.M., "Methionine Adenosyltransferase and S-Adenosylmethionine in the Developing Rat Lens" *Experimental Eye Research* (August 1988): 47 (2): 197-204.
4. Gharib, A., Sarda, N., Chabannes, B., Cronenberger, L., and Pacheco, H., "The Regional Concentrations of S-Adenosyl-L-Methionine, S-Adenosyl-L-Homocysteine, and Adenosine in Rat Brain" *Journal of Neurochemistry* (March 1982): 38 (3): 810-5.
5. Varela-Morieras, G., Perez-Olleros, L., Garcia-Cuevas, M., and Ruiz-Roso, B., "Effects of Aging on Folate Metabolism in Rats Fed a Long-Term Folate Deficient Diet" *International Journal for Vitamin & Nutrition Research* (1994): 64 (4): 294-9.
6. Surtees, R., and Hyland, K., "Cerebrospinal Fluid Concentrations of S-Adenosylmethionine, Methionine, and 5-Methyltetrahydrofolate in a Reference Population: Cerebrospinal Fluid S-Adenosylmethionine Declines with Age in Humans" *Biochemical Medicine & Metabolic Biology* (October 1990): 44 (2): 192-9.
7. Morrison, L.D., Smith, D.D., and Kish, S.J., "Brain S-Adenosylmethionine Levels Are Severely Decreased in Alzheimer's Disease" *Journal of Neurochemistry* (September 1996): 57 (3): 1328-31.
8. Stramentinoli, G., Gualano, M., Catto, E., and Algeri, S., "Tissue Levels of S-Adenosylmethionine in Aging Rats" *Journal of Gerontology* (July 1977): 32 (4): 392-4.
9. Muccioli, G., Scordamaglia, A., Bertacco, S., and Dicarlo, R., "Effect of S-Adenosyl-L-Methionine on Brain Muscarinic Receptors of Aged Rats" *European Journal of Pharmacology* (2 November 1992): 227 (3): 293-9.
10. Muccioli, G., and Dicarlo, R., "S-Adenosyl-L-Methionine Restores Prolactin Receptors in the Aged Rabbit Brain" *European Journal of Pharmacology* (18 July 1989): 166 (2): 223-30.
11. Cimino, M., Vantini, G., Algeri, S., Curatola, G., Pezzoli, C., and Stramentinoli, G., "Age-Related Modifications of Dopaminergic and Beta-Adrenergic Receptor System: Restoration to Normal Activity by Modifying Membrane Fluidity with S-Adenosylmethionine" *Life Sciences* (21 May 1984): 34 (21): 2029-39.
12. Ando S., Tanaka, Y., Ono, Y., and Kon, K., "Incorporation Rate of Gm1 Ganglioside into Mouse Brain Myelin: Effect of Aging and Modification by Hormones and Other Compounds" *Advances in Experimental Medicine & Biology* (1984): 174: 241-8.

Chapter 15

1. Park, J., Tai, J., Roessner, C.A., and Scott, A.R., "Enzymatic Synthesis of S-Adenosyl-L-Methionine on the Preparative Scale" *Bioorganic and Medicinal Chemistry* (December 1996): 4 (12): 2179-85.
2. Fiecchi, A., *Sulfonic Acid Salts of S-Adenosilmethionine.* U.S. Patent No. 4,057,686. (8 November 1977).
3. Fiecchi, A., *Double Salts of S-Adenosil-L-Methionine* U.S. Patent No. 3,954,726. (4 May 1976).

GLOSSARY

ACTH Adrenocorticotropic hormone, a normal by-product of the pituitary gland. Its function is to regulate production of the adrenal hormone cortisol.

Acupuncture A practice, originally Chinese, involving inserting a needle at specific points of the body to cure disease or relieve pain.

Addison's Disease A rare endocrine disease that results from the diminished output of the hormones aldosterone and cortisol by the adrenal glands. Symptoms include weakness, low blood pressure, anemia, low blood sugar, and electrolyte abnormalities.

Agonist A substance that enhances a process. (Compare with antagonist.)

Alzheimer's Disease A form of senility caused by destruction (decay) of the frontal lobes of the brain, which leads to the progressive deterioration of mental function.

Amino Acid An organic acid containing an amino group (NH2). Amino acids are the end-product of protein metabolism.

ANA A group of antibodies that react against contents of the cell nucleus. These antibodies are present in a variety of immunologic diseases.

Antidepressant A group of medications intended to decrease the symptoms associated with depression.

Anti-inflammatory A substance that decreases the signs and symptoms (pain and swelling) of inflammation.

Antioxidant A chemical that decreases or prevents the breakdown of fatty acids within tissues. Vitamin C is an antioxidant.

Arrhythmia A disturbance of the heart's beat or consistency.

Arthroscopy A procedure involving the insertion of a thin fiberoptic scope into a joint space in order to view its internal structures. Sometimes surgery can also be performed using an arthroscope.

Ascites A collection of fluid in the abdomen, usually as a result of increased pressure in the portal system due to liver obstruction. It can also be caused by cancer or intra-abdominal inflammation.

ATP Adenosine tri-phosphate, a molecule used in the cells of the body to store energy.

Bio-active Capable of having an effect on a living organism.

Bio-availability The extent to which a substance is available to the body. For example, calcium gluconate delivers more calcium to where it is needed than calcium carbonate, and is thus is more bio-available.

Bradykinesia Slowed body movements.

BUN Blood urea nitrogen, a measure of either kidney function or red blood cell destruction.

Cardiac Something near to, affecting, about, or in the heart.

Cartilage A tough connective tissue that forms joints and provides a structure for the nose and ears.

Catecholamine A neurotransmitter that causes excitatory responses in the brain and body. Examples include epinephrine and norepinephrine.

Glossary

CBC Complete blood count, a general measure of the cells in the blood. It can identify infection, anemia, and other conditions. It also describes some of the characteristics of red blood cells, such as their size and hemoglobin content.

Chemical Depression A notion that depression is the result of a deficiency or imbalance in brain transmitters or hormones.

Chemotherapy Chemotherapeutic agents are medications used to treat a variety of cancers. These medications are given in a specific regimen over a period of weeks.

Chiropractic A healing practice based on the science of the relationship between the spinal column and nervous system.

Chondrocyte A cartilage cell. Chondrocytes are the only living component of cartilage.

Chondroitin Sulfate A primary component of the external cellular form and connective tissue of animals, found on the outside of the cell membranes of some animal cells.

Chondromalacia The gradual erosion of cartilage, common in the knee joint where it is known as chondromalacia patella.

Chondroprotective A substance that either does not destroy or actually helps to build cartilage.

Cirrhosis An irreversible tissue change in the liver as a result of severe damage due to the effects of alcohol, viruses, or other toxins.

Collagen A structural protein involved in the development of connective tissue.

Crepitance A crackling sound that occurs in arthritic joints.

CT Scan Computerized axial tomography (CT), a special radiographic procedure that uses a computer to blend multiple x-ray images. CT scans can reveal many soft tissue structures not detectable by conventional x-rays.

Cushing's Disease An increased blood concentration of glucocorticoid hormone (produced by the adrenal gland). It results from a pituitary tumor that secretes the hormone adrenocorticotropic hormone (ACTH), which stimulates the adrenal gland to produce excess glucocorticoids.

Degenerative Disease A disease that, once it starts, grows progressively more severe. Parkinson's disease, cirrhosis of the liver, osteoarthritis, and Alzheimer's disease are all degenerative diseases.

Delusion A false belief or beliefs, most often seen in psychosis.

Depression A clinical affliction characterized by a persistent sad mood and/or loss of interest in activities. Signs of depression include changes in eating habits, insomnia, early morning wakening, apathy, depressed mood, fatigue, and suicidal thoughts.

Detoxification The process of removing a poisonous substance or changing it to an inert one.

DHEA Di-hydro-epi-andosterone, a hormone produced by the adrenal glands.

DNA Deoxyribonucleic acid, a material in the chromosomes of cell nuclei that contains the genetic code.

Double-blind Study A scientific experiment in which neither the experimenter nor the subjects know what substance the subjects are receiving.

Echinacea An herb commonly used for maintaining the immune system.

Edema Swelling that occurs due to an overaccumulation of fluid in body tissues.

Glossary

Electromyography (EMG)   A process that measures the electrical currents of a muscle.

Epithelium   The thin cell layer covering all membranes, especially the skin.

ESR   Sedimentation rate, a test that measures the rate of fall of red blood cells in a tube. It is a general measure of inflammation.

Fat Soluble   A substance that dissolves in fat. Some vitamins, such as vitamin E, are fat soluble.

Fiberoptics   A flexible fiberoptic scope that is used to see the internal anatomy of a hollow organ.

Fibromyalgia   A disorder characterized by muscle pain, stiffness, and fatigue.

Foxglove   A flowering herb that is the source of digitalis.

GI   Gastrointestinal; connected to or communicating with the stomach and intestine.

Glucosamine   An amino sugar (2 amino 2 deoxyglucose). It is a component of chitin, heparan sulfate, chondroitin sulfate, and many complex polysaccharides.

Growth Hormone   A hormone that activates the growth of bones and muscles.

HAM-D   A test that tries to objectively measure the severity of depression.

Hemachromatosis   A disease characterized by the proliferation of red blood cells.

HMO   Health Maintenance Organization. A medical insurance organization with subscriber physicians and patients, designed to regulate medical costs.

Homeopathy   A system of medical practice that treats a disease with small amounts of a substance that is known to cause symptoms similar to those of the disease in healthy people.

Homocysteine   A sulfur-containing amino acid. There is some suggestion that homocysteine is a beneficial substance in heart disease.

Hyperalertness (hypervigilance)   An emotional state in which a person is unable to relax. It leads to myalgias, anxiety, and depression. Often a person is so accustomed to being in this state, he is not aware of it.

Hypertension   An above-normal systolic or diastolic blood pressure. This condition is considered a risk factor for the development of heart disease, peripheral vascular disease, stroke, and kidney disease.

Hypokinesia   Decreased muscular activity.

Insulin   A hormone produced by the pancreas. Insulin controls the body's metabolism of glucose and is necessary for cells to absorb glucose in order to produce energy.

Intracellular   Present, occurring, or working within a cell.

Intraduodenal   Bypassing the stomach.

Leukemia   A blood disease in which the white blood cells are abnormal in type and/or number.

Libido   Emotional or psychic energy that in psychoanalytic theory is derived from primitive biological urges and is usually goal-directed.

Ligament   Strong connective tissue that serves to stabilize joints.

Limbic System   A poorly understood web of neurons in the central nervous system that seems to relate to activities such as waking and sleeping.

L-Tryptophan   An essential amino acid thought to be beneficial in relieving anxiety states.

Glossary

MAO inhibitor   A drug that blocks monoamine oxidase (MAO), an enzyme that is produced in the brain and the liver. MAO is involved in breaking down norepinephrine, serotonin, and dopamine. Therefore, inhibiting its action helps maintain higher levels of these neurotransmitters.

Melatonin   A hormone produced at night by the pineal gland (located at the center of the brain). It is believed to control the body's biological clock and reproductive cycles.

Meta-analysis   A study that combines similar aspects of several smaller studies. It is designed to provide a wider sample than any of the individual studies would be able to achieve.

Metabolism   The process by which substances are broken down into simpler substances or waste products, thereby releasing the energy needed for body functions.

Methionine   A crystalline sulfur-containing essential amino acid with the formula $C_5H_{11}NO_2S$. It is a precursor to SAMe.

Methyl Donor   A substance that gives off a methyl group (CH_3) in a chemical reaction known as methylation.

Migraine   A recurring form of headache. Migraines are identified by uneven throbbing headaches that are accompanied by nausea, vomiting, and sensitivity to light.

MRI   A diagnostic method that produces computerized images of internal body tissues. It is based on nuclear magnetic resonance of atoms within the body, which are induced by the application of radio waves.

Myofascial Pain Syndrome   A syndrome characterized by localized pain and the presence of trigger points, which when pressed refer pain to a different site.

Naturopathy   A system of disease treatment that avoids drugs and surgery and emphasizes the use of natural agents like air, water, and sunshine, or physical means like manipulation and electrical treatment.

Neurotransmitter   A chemical substance that is released from the axon terminal of a nerve cell to influence another nerve cell. Examples include serotonin, norepinephrine, and dopamine.

NSAID   Nonsteroidal anti-inflammatory. Any of several related drugs used to reduce inflammation and relieve pain.

Osmolality   The concentration of particles in water.

Osteoarthritis   A form of arthritis that results in degeneration of the articular surfaces (synovium) of the joints.

Palpitations   A sensation that the heart is beating very fast.

Pancreatitis   An inflammation of the pancreas.

Parkinson's Disease   A neurological disease first described in 1817 by James Parkinson. The pathology is not completely understood, but it appears to involve consistent changes in the melanin-containing nerve cells in the brain stem (substantia nigra, locus coeruleus), leading to a progressive inability to initiate voluntary movements and a corresponding increase in involuntary movements.

Patellofemoral Syndrome (PFS)   Chondromalacia, a painful condition of the knee brought on by disrupted patellar (kneecap) cartilage and poor conditioning of the knee.

pH   The concentration of hydrogen ions in a liquid. The greater the concentration, the lower the pH and the more acidic the solution. pH numbers in-

Glossary

crease exponentially; thus a pH of 5 has 10 times more hydrogen atoms (and is five times more acidic) than a pH of 6. The average pH of the body is 7.4.

PNI Psychoneuroimmunology. The field of science that correlates the processes of mind and body.

Polycythemia Vera A disease of unknown cause that produces more red blood cells than are necessary for the body to function.

Prostaglandins Any of a class of physiologically active substances present in many tissues, with effects such as vasodilation, vasoconstriction, stimulation of intestinal or bronchial smooth muscle, uterine contractions, and antagonism to hormones influencing lipid metabolism.

Protein Any of numerous, naturally occurring, extremely complex substances that consist of amino-acid residues joined by peptide bonds and contain the elements carbon, hydrogen, nitrogen, oxygen, usually sulfur, and occasionally other elements (such as phosphorus or iron). Proteins include many essential biological compounds, such as enzymes, hormones, and immunoglobulins.

Proteoglycan A complex of protein and polysaccharide, characteristic of the structural tissues of vertebrates, such as bone and cartilage, but also present on cell surfaces. It is important in determining viscoelastic properties of joints and other structures subject to mechanical deformation.

Prozac (fluoxetine) A common prescription anti-depressant drug. Prozac is classed as a selective serotonin re-uptake inhibitor, or SSRI, which functionally means that it increases the levels of serotonin in the body.

Psychotherapy The treatment of mental or emotional disorders or of related bodily ills by psychological means.

Radical A group of atoms that acts as a single atom in chemical reactions.

Retin-A This brand name for tretinoin, a drug used to treat acne and decrease wrinkles. It works partly by keeping skin pores clear.

Rheumatoid Arthritis (RA) A systemic disease, seen more commonly in women, that affects connective tissue, particularly the synovial tissue within joints.

Rheumatology A medical science dealing with rheumatic diseases (that is, diseases that affect connective tissue).

RNA Ribonucleic acid; a genetic code for proteins.

Serotonin A neurotransmitter found in the central nervous system. Serotonin is also released by blood platelets after injury. Together with histamine, serotonin plays a role in mediating allergic reactions and the inflammatory response.

Single-blind Study A scientific experiment in which the experimenter, but not the subjects, knows what substance each subject is receiving.

St. John's wort An herb used to treat depression.

Steroid A hormone with a cholesterol-base molecule, made in the body and used to control metabolic and sexual functioning.

Synovium The lining of a joint.

Synthetase An enzyme that synthesizes (creates) a specific substance. SAMe synthetase synthesizes SAMe from methionine and ATP.

Tagamet One of a class of anti-ulcer medication(s) that work by inhibiting the secretion of gastric acids. Examples include cimetidine (Tagamet), famotidine (Pepcid), nizatidine (Axid), and ranitidine (Zantac).

Glossary

Tai Chi   An ancient Chinese discipline of meditative movements practiced as a system of exercises.

Temporomandibular Joint   The joint that connects the lower jaw to the skull.

TENS Unit   Transcutaneous electrical nerve stimulation unit. A device used to relieve pain by delivering low level electrical stimulation to the painful area.

Uncontrolled Study   A scientific experiment in which both the experimenter and the subjects are aware of the treatment being given.

Uric Acid   A substance formed in the breakdown of nucleoproteins in the tissues, and excreted in the urine.

Wilson's Disease   An inborn disease that prevents copper from being metabolized, thus allowing it to damage the liver, resulting in cirrhosis.

INDEX

Index